D1542197

BASICS OF GROUP PSYCHOTHERAPY

BASICS
OF GROUP
PSYCHOTHERAPY

Edited by
Harold S. Bernard
K. Roy MacKenzie

THE GUILFORD PRESS
New York   London

© 1994 The Guilford Press
A Division of Guilford Publications, Inc.
72 Spring Street, New York, NY 10012

Printed in the United States of America

This book is printed on acid-free paper.

Last digit is print number: 9   8   7   6   5   4   3

Library of Congress Cataloging-in-Publication Data

Basics of group psychotherapy / edited by Harold S. Bernard,
   K. Roy MacKenzie,
     p. cm.
   Includes bibliographical references and index.
   ISBN 0-89862-117-8
   1. Group psychotherapy—Handbooks, manuals, etc.
I. Bernard, Harold S. II. MacKenzie, K. Roy, 1937–
   [DNLM: 1. Psychotherapy, Group. WM430 M294 1994]
RC488.M32 1994
616.89'152—dc20
DNLM/DLC
for Library of Congress   94-16964
                                     CIP

CONTRIBUTORS

Harold S. Bernard, Ph.D., Clinical Associate Professor of Psychiatry and Chief, Group Psychotherapy Program, Division of Ambulatory Services, New York University/Bellevue Medical Center, New York, New York

Robert R. Dies, Ph.D., Professor of Psychology, University of Maryland, College Park, Maryland

Elaine Cooper Lonergan, M.S.W., Ph.D., Associate Clinical Professor and Associate Director of Group Therapy Training, Department of Psychiatry, University of California at San Francisco School of Medicine, San Francisco, California

K. Roy MacKenzie, M.D., Clinical Professor of Psychiatry, University of British Columbia, Vancouver, British Columbia, Canada

Mary McCallum, Ph.D., Assistant Clinical Professor, Department of Psychiatry, University of Alberta, Edmonton, Alberta, Canada

William E. Piper, Ph.D., Professor, Department of Psychiatry, University of Alberta, Edmonton, Alberta, Canada

Kenneth Porter, M.D., Assistant Clinical Professor of Psychiatry, Columbia College of Physicians and Surgeons, New York, New York

Judith Schoenholtz-Read, Ed.D., [formerly Lazerson], Associate Dean in Clinical Psychology, The Fielding Institute, Santa Barbara, California

PREFACE

This book is addressed to clinicians both in training and in practice who are beginning, or at least beginning to consider, utilizing group psychotherapy as part of their "armamentarium." Our intent is to focus on specific skills—on the nuts-and-bolts issues involved in running therapy groups. It is designed as a complementary volume to the standard group psychotherapy textbook. The book is organized as you would organize a group, beginning with the selection of patients for the particular group, followed by an introduction to the idea of group development. The next three chapters deal with the struggles confronted and opportunities available to the leaders of therapy groups. The sixth chapter offers an overview of the variety of groups available today, including nontherapy groups. Finally, the last chapter explicates the range of different theories that pertain to treatment groups. This sequence is the opposite of most books on psychotherapy, in which the emphasis is heavily on theory from the outset.

We have tried to focus on what you, as a relatively new group psychotherapist, actually need to do. Above all, this book is concerned with how you as a therapist can make your groups most effective. This means stepping back and conceptualizing yourself as providing therapy *through* the group, not through interaction with individual patients.

Group psychotherapy requires additional skills that are not learned through training and experience in individual psychotherapy. The most important additional skill or sensibility is the ability to conceptualize the entire group as a system, which is in some ways parallel to the paradigm shift required to do family therapy. All group therapists feel the pull from time to time to do individual therapy in the group setting, and many patients expect it. Resisting such a pull is an ongoing task for the therapist.

The therapy group is a vehicle for enacting, and thus for potentially understanding, how things unfold in participants' interpersonal worlds. To facilitate this, the skilled therapist will constantly try to ensure interaction among the members, followed by reflection on what that interaction reveals. This process is particularly important in the early stages of a group, when the preeminent task is to promote the development of group cohesion. It is analogous to the "therapeutic alliance" in individual therapy because it is a precondition for effective therapy.

Over the last decade and a half, there has been a concerted effort to demonstrate that psychotherapy is effective. Hundreds of controlled studies are now available that indicate an overall therapeutic effect of about 0.85; that is, about 85% of patients receiving psychotherapy do significantly better than control group patients. That the results are essentially the same whether the psychotherapy is delivered in an individual or group format is not well known. For this reason, among others, there is currently a great deal of interest in the use of group therapy. Groups offer a considerable advantage of efficiency, and treatment outcome seems to be comparable. In addition, time line studies show that the majority of patients achieve positive results in a relatively short period of time—usually measured in months. Longer-term groups therefore are increasingly likely to be used for severely dysfunctional patients only.

Group psychotherapy can be thought of as a treatment modality through which a wide variety of different types of therapy can be offered. In Chapter 1, Piper and McCallum describe a very careful approach to patient selection which is clearly and integrally tied to the nature of the group the therapist intends to conduct. An effective group is usually one where the particular approach taken has been carefully thought through, and patients who can potentially benefit from the approach decided upon have been carefully selected. To put this another way, the phrase "group psychotherapy" is not very informative. It describes the structure but not the content of the therapy.

Another important perspective on making sense of group events is that of developmental stages. An understanding of these stages allows the therapist to think ahead to what is likely to happen and, therefore, to be in a position to detect early indications and reinforce them. In Chapter 2, MacKenzie describes a sequence common to all groups that consists of four stages of development and delineates the tasks and issues that must be attended to in each.

Chapters 3 through 5 are devoted to various aspects of the complex challenge of group leadership. In Chapter 3, Dies provides a comprehensive description of specific leadership tasks and skills. In Chapter 4, Porter explicates some of the basic concerns of all group therapists: transference, resistance, countertransference, and the emergence of primitive group dynamics. He also addresses the vexing but seldom discussed matter of the negative effect a group can have for some participants—a reality in all forms of psychotherapy that can be minimized with training and skill, but never eliminated. In Chapter 5, Bernard describes a variety of problematic patients and situations that group therapists frequently confront and suggests concrete strategies for dealing with them.

In Chapter 6, Schoenholtz-Read gives a thorough overview of the enormous variety of groups available to "consumers." She offers criteria for helping therapists, who have determined that some kind of group intervention is desirable for a particular individual, to choose the most appropriate kind of group experience for their client.

The final chapter, placed at the end of the book intentionally, provides a concise overview of the major theories that have been developed to help leaders understand group processes. Group theory often makes dry, if not incomprehensible, reading until one has actually experienced the group milieu. The pressures that build in a group can be elusive, unmistakable but often difficult to describe. This chapter provides some concepts for understanding and attempting to address such group-level phenomena.

Our hope is that this book will encourage readers to undertake, or go further with, the work of conducting psychotherapy groups. While groups can be complicated and even overwhelming at times, they can also be extremely exciting: Groups can make a real difference in the lives of those who participate in them, and can be very gratifying for therapists to conduct. For these reasons, we have come to devote a great deal of our professional energies to running groups, teaching others to do the same, and writing about what we have learned. We hope this volume helps to make you as enthusiastic about the enterprise of group psychotherapy as we are.

HAROLD S. BERNARD
K. ROY MACKENZIE

CONTENTS

ONE • **SELECTION OF PATIENTS**   1
FOR GROUP INTERVENTIONS
William E. Piper and Mary McCallum

General Selection Criteria for Group Therapy, 2
Aspects of the Group and
   Patient Selection Criteria, 6
Forms of Group Therapy and Patient Selection, 11
Special Assessment Procedures, 22
Training in Patient Selection, 28
Conclusion, 29

TWO • **THE DEVELOPING STRUCTURE**   35
OF THE THERAPY GROUP SYSTEM
K. Roy MacKenzie

Engagement Stage, 36
Differentiation Stage, 47
The Working Group, 53
Termination Stage, 57
Conclusion, 58

THREE • **THE THERAPIST'S ROLE IN GROUP TREATMENTS**   60
Robert R. Dies

Pregroup Preparation, 63
Early Group Sessions, 65
Transition Period, 74
Working Sessions, 82
Termination, 93
Conclusion, 96

FOUR • **PRINCIPLES OF GROUP**   100
THERAPEUTIC TECHNIQUE
Kenneth Porter

General Principles of Group Leadership, 101
Resistance, 103

Transference, 107
Primitive Group Dynamics, 112
Countertransference, 115
Negative Effects of Group Therapy, 119
Conclusion, 122

FIVE ● **DIFFICULT PATIENTS** 123
AND CHALLENGING SITUATIONS
Harold S. Bernard

Difficult Patients, 125
Challenging Situations, 137
Conclusion, 156

SIX ● **SELECTION OF GROUP INTERVENTION** 157
Judith Schoenholtz-Read

Common Characteristics of Helping Groups, 160
Group Interventions for Patients with
    Severe Problems, 165
Group Interventions for Patients
    with Moderate Problems, 170
Group Interventions for Moderate
    to Mild Problems, 180
Combining Psychotherapy and
    "Other-than-Therapy" Groups, 183
Conclusion, 185

SEVEN ● **USING THEORIES OF GROUP THERAPY** 189
Elaine Cooper Lonergan

The Therapy Session, 191
Freud's Group Psychology, 193
Basic Assumption Theory, 196
Group Focal Conflict Theory, 198
Living Systems Theory, 200
Foulkes's Psychoanalysis in Groups, 204
Yalom's Here-and-Now Approach, 207
Cognitive-Behavioral Approach, 209
Conclusion, 214

● **INDEX** 217

BASICS OF GROUP PSYCHOTHERAPY

• ONE •

SELECTION OF PATIENTS FOR GROUP INTERVENTIONS

William E. Piper
Mary McCallum

Yalom (1975) stated that "the fate of a therapy group and its members is to a large extent determined before the first group session" (p. 19). His observation emphasizes the importance of patient selection to successful experiences in therapy groups. Patient selection involves making decisions about whether particular patients should be included in a group or excluded from it. Clinicians routinely decide whether to refer patients to group therapy, individual therapy, or alternatives, including no therapy. Their decision requires a consideration of qualities that patients presumably must possess to remain, work, and benefit in therapy groups. Such qualities constitute patient selection criteria.

The notion of a relation between patient selection criteria and successful group experiences is hardly new to clinicians or researchers. A number of general selection criteria believed to be relevant for all forms of group therapy have been proposed in the clinical literature. More recently, the trend has been toward matching specific selection criteria with particular forms of group therapy. That trend reflects the idea that characteristics of groups, for example, theoretical approaches, goals, and techniques, have implications for the type of patients that should be selected. Whereas this approach promises fewer selection failures, it probably cannot be expected to guarantee "failsafe" selection criteria. Therapy

1

groups challenge patients to change in important ways, so it is likely that some patients will always become intimidated or discouraged and decide against continuing treatment. In addition, many therapists prefer to admit some "risky" patients, reasoning that potential gains outweigh potential risks and that the patient is entitled to an opportunity to benefit. Even for those therapists who accept only "safe" candidates, the factors involved in selection decisions are complex and difficult to identify and quantify. Nevertheless, the more we can identify suitable candidates for group therapy, the more we can prevent the demoralizing effects for patients and therapists that are associated with failures and casualties.

In this chapter, we review the clinical and research literature concerning patient selection criteria for group psychotherapy. First we summarize general selection criteria that have been proposed. Next we consider the suggestion that particular treatment approaches require specific patient selection criteria. For purposes of illustration we present and consider the relationships between two particular treatment approaches (long-term, time-unlimited, supportive group psychotherapy and short-term, time-limited, interpretive group psychotherapy) and two specific selection criteria (psychological mindedness and quality of object relations). Additional selection criteria for the two types of treatment are also considered. Finally training in patient selection is addressed.

GENERAL SELECTION CRITERIA FOR GROUP THERAPY

Friedman (1976) identified three approaches to patient selection: nonlegitimate, illegitimate, and legitimate. The nonlegitimate approach is when the referral does not reflect a consideration of the needs of the patient. Referring a patient to a group for student training purposes is an example of a nonlegitimate approach. The illegitimate approach is when the referral stems from the referring therapist's negative reaction to the patient. For example, the therapist may dislike the patient and transfer him or her to the group therapist.

The legitimate approach to patient selection is when the referring therapist considers group therapy as the treatment of choice for the patient. A legitimate approach to the formulation of selection criteria requires an attitude that views group therapy not as a second-class treatment but as a unique treatment from which certain patients in particular may benefit. Given that approach, authors such as Grunebaum and Kates (1977), Sadock (1983), and Klein (1983) recommend for group therapy patients who experience difficulties in their interpersonal relationships, for example, patients whose relationships are characterized by withdrawal, overdependency, or a pattern of multiple and transient encounters. In addition, patients who have paranoid reactions to authority figures might benefit from group therapy; their paranoid reactions can diffuse and dissipate when confronted by the differing impressions of other group members. Interpersonal inhibitions of these patients, however, may be so intense that the patients are paralyzed in the group or scared away prematurely.

We should also note that given the unique opportunity to explore interpersonal relations afforded by group therapy, many clinicians believe it to be a useful adjunct to other types of therapy. The rationale for offering concurrent therapies is that different issues can be addressed by the different therapy formats. For example, marital issues can be best addressed in marital therapy, interpersonal issues in group therapy, and intrapersonal issues in individual therapy. The disadvantage of concurrent therapies is the potential risk of diluting the therapeutic impact of each therapy. For example, the patient may sit silently in group, saving up disclosures for his or her individual therapist. The need to discourage the dilution of therapy's impact may be particularly salient for a therapist practicing interpretive therapy. Conversely, a therapist practicing supportive therapy may encourage patients to expand their support network by participating in concurrent therapies.

An alternative approach to selection for group in comparison to individual therapy is choosing patients with greater interpersonal skills or capabilities. This selection rationale, however, can lead to a paradox in which those who are selected are those who are the least in need. Rather than accepting patients with particularly high or low interpersonal skills, Woods and Melnick (1979) suggested that the minimal skills necessary for effective participation should be the selection criteria. Clinicians have suggested several characteristics that represent general selection criteria for group therapy. They are presented in Table 1.1.

Rather than emphasizing inclusion criteria, however, clinicians have traditionally paid much more attention to exclusion criteria. As Yalom (1985) has noted, "Given a pool of patients, they determine that certain

TABLE 1.1. General Patient Selection Criteria for Group Therapy

* Minimum level of interpersonal skill
* Motivation for treatment
* Positive expectations of gain from therapy
* Current psychological discomfort
* An interpersonal problem
* Commitment to changing interpersonal behavior
* Susceptibility to the group influence (moderate approval-dependency)
* Willingness to be of help to others

ones cannot possibly work in a therapy group and should be excluded, and then proceed to accept all the other patients" (p. 228). Patients typically excluded have been those who are brain damaged, paranoid, hypochondriacal, drug dependent, psychotic, sociopathic, suicidal, deeply depressed, and in crisis. The common rationale is that such patients are likely to be viewed as deviants who do not share the objectives of the group and who are unable to participate in the required interpersonal process of the group.

Concerning selection criteria based on research evidence, our review of the group psychotherapy literature revealed a large number of clinical studies that attempted to predict outcome based on pretherapy patient characteristics. Given such a wealth of data, it is perhaps not surprising that many statistically significant relationships have been reported. Many of the findings make conceptual and clinical sense, for example, evidence supporting a relationship between motivation and desirable therapy process or between social skills and favorable outcome. Nevertheless, most reviewers have not been impressed by the research literature, and their lack of enthusiasm reflects problems associated with this area of research. First, the number of nonsignificant relationships far outweigh significant ones. Thus there is a strong possibility that many of the significant relationships are chance findings. Second, although many correlations were statistically significant, most were small in magnitude and therefore of questionable clinical importance. Third, there has been a lack of replication of findings.

An explanation for the weak empirical evidence for patient predictor variables was offered by Woods and Melnick (1979). They suggested that the dyadic intake interview has been one of the most commonly used but least useful methods of obtaining predictor scores. Similarly, they were not impressed with the use of various screening scales and psychological tests for selection purposes. Woods and Melnick further charged that formal diagnostic categories, personality profiles, or current adjustment levels have seldom been significantly related to remaining, working, or benefitting in group therapy. They recommended using behavioral and interpersonal variables of actual group behaviors, and these variables have proven to be better predictors of subsequent group therapy behavior (Goldstein, Heller, & Sechrest, 1966; Piper & Marrache, 1981). The advantage of using such variables involves the similarity between the selection procedure and the group experience. Patients gain an experiential understanding of what to expect in group therapy. Similarly, the therapist can observe the patients in a group situation before final decisions regarding the therapy group are made.

In most clinics intake workers and therapists share duties and thus both are familiar with the tasks of assessment and treatment. However, in private practice group therapists often depend on referral sources to select patients for them. Therefore, we believe that the usefulness of group screens to select appropriate patients and to exclude inappropriate patients is particularly salient for private practitioners. In this case, the group therapist has considerably less knowledge of the individual patients than the referral sources. He or she must decide in a relatively brief period of time whether the eight or nine patients can work together in a group. It would delay the start of the group and be extremely time consuming for the group therapist to spend a few sessions with each patient individually in order to obtain a history of the presenting complaints, diagnosis, and family history. It would also be redundant, since that information is typically available from the referring agent. In addition, individual sessions may impede members' cohesion to the group or to the other patients relative to the leader.

The group therapist needs experiential knowledge of the patient's ability to work in a group and with the therapist in the group situation. The group screen can provide this type of experiential knowledge. Screening groups can be conducted with three or four patients at a time. In this way the therapist has sufficient time to focus on the individual patient in the group screen if he or she needs to investigate a particular concern.

If the practitioner begins screening while the referral process is still in progress, the number of additional referrals that are required can be estimated and the process can be regulated in a smooth manner. This point emphasizes the importance of the group therapist's relationship with his or her referral sources. The group therapist needs to be able to communicate to the referral source exactly what he or she is looking for without discouraging the referral of borderline candidates. It is usually helpful for the group therapist to provide referring sources with a form that requests relevant information. For example, if the therapist is recruiting patients for a bereavement group, the referral form should provide a space for the referring agent to list the losses experienced by the patient. In this way, the referring agent will be thinking about the criterion of loss when selecting patients for the group. In addition, the group therapist should be available to answer questions and provide feedback concerning the appropriateness of referrals. It should also be noted that if a private practitioner repeats the work of the referring agent by assessing each patient individually, he or she risks offending the referral agent, who may feel that his or her judgment is being questioned. In addition, the patient may resent having to pay for repetitive assessment sessions.

While we believe that screening groups are cost effective, some clinicians may regard the time and energy such groups require as a disadvantage. To gain more from the investment of time the screening process may be combined with preparations procedures. In this way two tasks can be accomplished simultaneously. Preparation has been shown to improve attendance, retention, and certain types of therapy process (Budman, Clifford, Bader, & Bader, 1981; Piper, Debbane, Bienvenu, & Garant, 1982; Piper & Perrault, 1989). If patients are well prepared for the group experience, they usually feel less anxious, disappointed, and dissatisfied in the group. Ideally they will feel that they "fit" in the group and be able to work more quickly, given their awareness of the task. Preparation thus has implications for patient selection. The referrer's selection criteria can be less stringent if patients are screened again as part of the preparation procedures that precede the therapy group.

The fact that preparation procedures can influence selection decisions argues against the assumption that a single client predictor, behavioral or otherwise, can be so powerful as to override other aspects of the group. However, prior research endeavours have been criticized for following that very approach. In the words of Roback and Smith (1987), "We believe that dropping out of treatment is usually a complex interaction between patient, group and therapist factors, but much of the literature tends to focus on only one of these dimensions" (p. 427). The interplay of these other dimensions are considered in the next section.

ASPECTS OF THE GROUP AND PATIENT SELECTION CRITERIA

The selection criteria the therapist uses are governed by several aspects of the group. These include the goals for the group, the theoretical approach, the therapist technique, the strategy for composing the group, and structural aspects of the group. The influence of the interplay of these various aspects of the group on selection criteria suggests that patients deemed suitable for one type of group therapy may not be suitable for other types of group therapy.

Group Approach and Goals

To illustrate how multiple aspects of the group influence patient selection criteria, consider the following example. Assume that you decide to conduct an inpatient therapy group with the objective of decreasing recidivism. Because the hospital provides a safe atmosphere in which patients can be contained and observed after group, you need not exclude suicidal or psychotic patients. Assume that your theoretical orientation is biochemical, that is, you believe that you can reduce recidivism by increasing patients' compliance with taking medications. Your theoretical orientation will influence your plans for technique and the structural aspects of the group, which in turn will influence patient selection. Given your biochemical theoretical orientation, your technique emphasizes providing information in a didactic way regarding the dosage levels and side effects of medication: You exclude psychotic patients who will be confused in the group. Given your didactic technique, you decide to compose a homogeneous group according to a target diagnosis that responds well to medication: You select patients according to your target diagnosis. Your technique suggests that the membership be closed so that you need not repeat information to newcomers: You select patients who are available for all group sessions. Due to the relatively brief duration of most hospitalizations, the group is short-term and time-limited, for example, two or three sessions during the week prior to discharge: You select patients who are ready for discharge. Toward your goal of reducing recidivism by discussing the merits of continuing medication, you form a homogeneous group of four predischarge patients who are recovering from a manic episode.

Let us next consider how the patient selection criteria would be affected by a different theoretical approach. Your objective is still to decrease recidivism, but assume that your theoretical orientation is cognitive-behavioral. You believe that you can best achieve your goal by helping patients recognize anxiety-inducing situations and then evaluate and respond to those situations more effectively. You further believe that patients can achieve these changes in recognition, evaluation, and response style by changing the cognitions that occur in response to stress. Your technique would reflect your theoretical orientation in that you would want to engage in providing corrective information, self-reinforcement training, cognitive restructuring, and self-instructional training (Rose, 1990; Yost, Beutler, Corbishley, & Allender, 1986).

In terms of patient selection, you exclude psychotic patients who would be confused in the group. Since your technique involves modeling and instructing alternate ways of responding, you exclude those who do not actively participate on the ward. Given that you believe that particular manifestations of psychopathology, such as depression, reflect characteristic, ineffectual cognitive processes, you employ a homogeneous composition strategy according to a target diagnosis: You select patients according to your target diagnosis. Your technique suggests that the membership should be closed so that you can avoid repeating phases of therapy for newcomers. Thus, you select patients who are available for all group sessions. Due to the relatively brief duration of most hospitalizations, the group is short-term and time-limited, for example, two or three sessions per week for two or three weeks. You select patients who have been stabilized on medications but who will not be discharged for another few weeks. Toward your goal of reducing recidivism by addressing the cognitive processes of inpatients and by modeling and instructing alternate ways of responding, you form a homogeneous group of four available patients who have been diagnosed with depression.

Considering yet a third example, assume that your theoretical approach is existential. You believe that you can best achieve your goal by minimizing patients' social isolation and alienation. This change in theoretical orientation will change your plans for therapist technique and the structural aspects of the group, which in turn will change your patient selection criteria. Given your existential theoretical orientation, your technique emphasizes facilitating and supporting the expression of universal fears among members. Consistent with this technique, you employ a heterogeneous composition strategy. You do not exclude any patient. The technique encourages the instillation of hope. Membership is open to all patients who wish to participate, even after discharge. To accommodate competing ward activities for hospitalized patients and competing schedules for discharged patients, the group is held once weekly for one hour. Given the broad objective and flexible structure, the selection criteria are broad. Patients join the group as soon as they want, attend as frequently or infrequently as they deem necessary, and may continue after discharge. The size of the group can vary from 5 to 25 patients.

The goals of a therapy group are strong determinants of patient selection criteria. It is also true that certain goals are more consistent with particular theoretical approaches than others and that they are better achieved utilizing particular therapist techniques within a specific group structure. However, as our examples demonstrate, the theoretical approach is primary in influencing patient selection criteria. It directly influences plans for the technique, which in turn influences the group's structure, the composition strategy, and ultimately the patient selection criteria. It is important, therefore, for the group therapist to be clear about his or her theoretical orientation.

There are many theoretical orientations: inspirational–supportive, didactic, confrontational, actionistic, psychodramatic, Gestalt, behavioral, cognitive, existential–supportive, and psychodynamic. Once affiliated with a theoretical approach, other aspects of the group, including patient selection criteria, logically follow in a manner consistent with the approach. The next section briefly summarizes selection issues that are associated with other aspects.

Therapist Factors

An example of how a therapist factor affected selection criteria was described by Martin Grotjahn (1972). Apparently frustrated with the selection paradox in which the patients most in need of group therapy seem to be the least likely to receive it, Grotjahn made a concerted effort to give doubtful patients a chance in his own practice. Although many of these risky patients dropped out, Grotjahn maintained his conviction about giving such patients an opportunity to benefit. In a similar vein, after highlighting a number of contradictory positions on the types of patients deemed suitable for group therapy, Mullan and Rosenbaum (1975) voiced their impression that "as the group therapist gains experience, he will become less selective" (p. 425). Accordingly, therapist values and experience appear quite capable of influencing selection criteria.

Other related factors that may influence selection criteria are the volume of the therapist's caseload and the patient population with whom the therapist works. Given the time and cost required to provide individual therapy to a large volume of homogeneous patients, practitioners have begun experimenting with the more cost-effective group modality. As Bond and Lieberman (1978) noted, "Deviant behavior, whether it be delinquency, alcoholism, or child abuse, has been successfully approached in a variety of situations" (p. 682). This position reflects the growing recognition that there are few patients for whom some type of group is not appropriate. One should note that whether due to circumstances or to design, groups addressing the needs of particular "deviant" populations have tended to be homogeneously composed. Hence, as the selection criteria have been broadened, structural aspects of the group have required adaptation, emphasizing the interplay among all aspects of the group.

Group Composition

Decisions about which combination of patients work most effectively together influence group composition. The challenge is to determine which blend of individual member characteristics enhance a type of group interaction or process that results in positive outcomes for each individual member. Pragmatically, composition involves stipulating which patient characteristics, if any, should be shared by all group members. Hence, approaches to composition typically favor either homogeneous or heterogeneous membership. There are arguments that favor and arguments that oppose each approach. For example, homogeneously composed groups are believed to coalesce more quickly, offer more immediate support, and elicit better attendance. Hence, group maintenance is seen as a priority. Arguments that favor heterogeneous composition include the notion that the range of conflicts in group members offers more opportunity for interpersonal learning on a deeper level. In reality, the difference may be artificial. First, all homogeneously composed groups are heterogeneous in some dimensions. Second, all new groups, however heterogeneous, find shared characteristics to lower tension in the interest of group maintenance. Third, homogeneous group members may be able to interact around a single area with more depth and understanding than a heterogeneously composed group which examines several areas.

The composition strategy typically reflects the length of time over which the group will meet and the theoretical orientation of the therapist. Practitioners of long-term, dynamically oriented groups advocate that members be heterogeneous in terms of conflict content and defense mechanisms but homogeneous in their ability to tolerate anxiety and work. Long-term support groups tend to have homogeneous composition regarding a primary concern, for example, friends of schizophrenics. For short-term groups, regardless of theoretical orientation, homogeneous composition around a common presenting complaint is often recommended (MacKenzie, 1990). For short-term dynamically oriented groups, common unconscious conflicts are usually desirable.

Group Structure

Group structure refers to such aspects as the number of members admitted, the anticipated length of membership, whether membership is open or closed, and the frequency and duration of sessions. Group structure influences the commitment required of group members. Greater commitment is required when the membership is small, closed, and long-term and the sessions are frequent and of long duration. The degree of commitment required of group members reflects the context of the group as well as the group's theoretical orientation.

Given the brief nature of most hospitalizations, inpatient and partial hospitalization groups are usually short-term in nature. They may be held daily or a few times a week, but they generally last only for a few weeks. The length of sessions is typically shorter than outpatient groups, reflecting the difficulty of highly distressed patients in containing their anxiety. Regarding the size of group membership, inpatient groups typically vary depending on competing ward activities, which also indicates that the membership is typically open to whomever is available to attend.

Outpatient groups tend to be conducted on a less frequent basis but over a longer period of time. Structural aspects of outpatient groups primarily reflect their theoretical orientation. For example, patients joining psychodynamically oriented groups may need to commit only to weekly sessions, but that commitment is paramount. The importance of commitment is reflected by the expectation of weekly attendance, the closed membership, and the relatively small membership. A psychodynamic outpatient group usually has between 7 and 12 patients. More traditional psychodynamic therapists prefer between 7 and 9 members, believing that more than 9 prohibits in-depth explorations. They do acknowledge that the larger group permits a stronger socialization effect, which can be supportive. The consensus is that for psychodynamically oriented groups, 5 and 12 are the lower and upper limits.

With support groups there is usually not the same demand for commitment in terms of regular attendance or length of participation. Membership is often open and members need not attend every week. Groups utilizing a supportive orientation can tolerate larger numbers. That flexibility reflects their therapeutic goal of promoting ego strength rather than encouraging in-depth exploration of uncomfortable emotions.

FORMS OF GROUP THERAPY AND PATIENT SELECTION

In this section of the chapter, we examine two forms of group therapy. The first is based on a humanistic–supportive theoretical approach and the second is based on an interpretive theoretical approach. In addition to the theoretical orientation, the patient selection criteria will reflect a consideration of the structural and compositional aspects of the group as well as the therapist technique, and patient preparation procedures.

Long-Term, Time-Unlimited, Supportive Group Psychotherapy (LTSG)

The LTSG presented in this section was developed for a heterogeneous population of chronic psychiatric outpatients who repeatedly present in crisis, who are in need of support, and who tend to discontinue contact when the crisis is resolved.

Theoretical Orientation

The theoretical orientation of LTSG reflects a composite of the principles and assumptions of humanistic and object relations theorists. The difficulties experienced by LTSG patients are assumed to be related to conscious and unconscious conflicts concerning their relationships with others. While they may yearn for closeness and intimacy, past experience has taught them to mistrust others and to protect themselves by isolating themselves and withdrawing. They may unconsciously sabotage all relationships on which they feel they are becoming dependent. This pattern makes them feel lonely and alienated without a consistent source of support. The anxiety engendered by therapies that demand commitment causes this patient population to discontinue contact. Conversely, a flexible therapy contract and therapeutic approach that aims to reduce anxiety may better engage these patients. The use of mutual support to foster recovery among chronic psychiatric patients has been documented in the clinical literature (Sampath, Kingston, & Dhindsa, 1971; Rosenberg, 1984). The advantage of therapist-led groups over leaderless groups is the promotion of safety and the identification with the therapists' ability to cope (Wallace, 1983).

Objectives

The primary objective of LTSG is to provide chronic psychiatric patients a place where they can feel support and a sense of belonging. This primary objective consists of several more specific subgoals. The group aims to promote the exchange of (1) emotional and cognitive experiences, (2) problem-solving strategies, (3) information regarding the nature of psychiatric disorders, (4) information regarding medications, and (5) feedback regarding the impact of their behavior.

Therapist Technique

The therapists' technique reflects an attempt to promote an atmosphere of safety and mutual support. The therapists actively encourage and facilitate participation among members. They do not allow silences to become lengthy; they invite reluctant members to talk about their concerns. Additionally, they do not allow disruptive interactions to persist; they interrupt abusive members and suggest alternative ways of verbalizing their needs. Except for these "emergency" interventions, the therapists do not personally offer advice or support to individual members. They also discourage attempts to focus on the therapists. Rather, they comment on the group's discussion by emphasizing the similarities among the members, in particular shared emotional reactions. While psychodynamically informed, the therapists neither encourage nor interpret negative transference. Rather, they promote a positive transference to themselves, the group, and the institution.

Composition

The patients referred to LTSG are heterogeneous with respect to demographic characteristics, diagnosis, and use of medication. However, given the goal of diminishing alienation and isolation, each group is relatively homogeneous with respect to the interpersonal style of its members. For example, one group is composed of patients who exhibit primitive interpersonal styles. They develop blatantly self-destructive relationships with partners and employers. They often impulsively act out their anger, leading to a series of unstable relationships. Another group is composed of patients who are better able to tolerate anger and frustration. They tend to sustain relationships where they feel abused, exploited, and unappreciated. The group therapists assess the interpersonal style of a patient before accepting him or her for a particular group.

Group Structure

The groups meet once weekly for an hour. They are led by a cotherapy team. Membership is open and of unlimited duration. A patient who has been referred to a group can attend at any time. In an attempt to engage new members, patients are asked to attend at least the first four consecutive sessions. In addition, the entry of new members is restricted to 3 patients every other week. The total membership of the group approaches 200, but attendance at any particular group session typically ranges from 10 to 20 members.

Preparation

Patients are prepared individually by the referring clinician and again during a 1-hour pretherapy screening group session. During the screening session each patient is invited to express concerns and expectations about the group. The therapists who conduct the groups attend the screen and choose patients whom they believe fit their particular group. Patients whose conditions may have deteriorated since the initial assessment interview can be identified during the screening session and referred for a more appropriate treatment, for example, hospitalization.

Patient Selection Criteria

Given the characteristics of the long-term group described, the selection criteria can be broad and flexible. Following is an excerpt from an assessment interview of a patient considered suitable for LTSG.

ASSESSOR: I understand that you're thinking about getting into some type of therapy. Maybe you could tell me what has led you to this decision.

SALLY: Well, I've not been feeling well for many years and nothing seems to help. I'm really tired of not feeling well, and all these pills don't work.

A: You say "all these pills don't work." Which pills are those?

S: Oh, they've been all kinds: Surmontil, Elavil, Prozac, Zoloft. You name it.

A: So it sounds like you've been depressed. How long have you been treated for depression?

S: About 15 years; since my mother died. It comes and goes, but I've never felt happy since.

A: And you say the pills don't work. What happens?

S: Well, the side effects are just so bad.

A: You found that with the Prozac and Zoloft, too?

S: Yes. I don't like taking pills.

A: In terms of "talk" therapy, this is the first time you've thought about that?

S: No, my husband and I went to see a marriage counselor, but that was a waste of time.

A: It didn't help?

S: No, my husband is selfish. He just does what he wants. He never thinks about my feelings.

A: So your husband refused to continue?

S: Well, actually, he and the counselor ganged up on me. I didn't feel supported.

A: In terms of your goals for therapy this time, what are they?

S: I'm tired of feeling all alone, no one's there for me.

A: Do you think it would be helpful if you and your husband came in together?

S: Oh, he won't come in. He thinks it's such a waste of time. You see, he doesn't think he's got a problem. I'm the problem.

A: What problem does he see?

S: Oh, that I'm never satisfied; I nag him all the time; let's see, that I'm too emotional; that I want too much.

A: Does it ever get so bad that you think of leaving him?

S: (*Laughing*) Every day.

A: Have you ever left him?

S: Oh, no, I love him too much to ever leave him. And the children need their father. When I married it was for better or worse.

A: Do you ever worry that he'll leave you?

S: All the time. But he's got it too good.

A: So in terms of what therapy could help you with—could you try and put that into words?

S: So I wouldn't feel so alone. It's so hard being with kids all day. I miss adult company. It's not fair to burden the kids with all this. They don't understand.

A: No, they don't. Well, it sounds like you could use some support to cope with all the things in your life. You mentioned that it all began with your mother's death. You think it would help to talk about that?

S: Yeah, but that was a long time ago. I need help with feeling lonely today.

A: We have a group that meets once a week—

S: (*Interrupting*) Oh, I couldn't come every week. It's too hard to get babysitters.

A: It would be for an hour and a half for 12 weeks.

S: Oh, no, I couldn't do that. Couldn't I just see you when things are getting to me? You know, just when I need to talk.

A: Yes, you could, but it sounds like what you struggle with is feeling alone and that no one understands. I think it might be more helpful for you to meet with people, just like yourself, who have a hard time sometimes. You could meet and see how other people cope with husbands who aren't there for them and that sense of loneliness you feel.

S: Yeah, maybe, but I couldn't come every week.

A: You wouldn't have to. We have another group that is run every week for an hour. You'd be welcome to come every week but it's up to you; you're the boss; you use the group as you see fit for as long as you see fit.

S: Well, how does it work . . . ?

The preceding vignette illustrates many of the selection criteria for LTSG. They are presented in Table 1.2. In summary, the patient, Sally, has struggled with depression for 15 years (criterion 1). She has been treated with a number of antidepressants but has never persisted through the side effects even with the newer medications, which have relatively few side effects (criterion 2). Similarly, she terminated marriage counseling after only a few sessions (criterion 3). She cannot or will not commit to a time-limited therapy that demands weekly attendance (criterion 4). Her description of her marriage suggests the kind of dependent interpersonal style for which LTSG would be recommended (criterion 5).

TABLE 1.2. Patient Selection Criteria for Long-Term Supportive Group Therapy

- Chronic psychiatric history
- Pattern of noncompliance with or premature discontinuation of medication
- Recurring pattern of numerous presentations followed by noncompliance with or premature termination from therapy
- Inability to commit to ongoing therapy
- Interpersonal style consistent with other members of the group (e.g., dependent, primitive)

Patient Exclusion Criteria

For safety reasons, patients who are actively suicidal, homicidal, or psychotic are not accepted into LTSG.

Patient Population

Misunis, Feist, Thorkelsson, and McAuley (1990) investigated the nature of patients accepted into various interpersonal style groupings of LTSG. As an example, patients referred to a group with dependent interpersonal styles represented all socioeconomic and demographic categories. Sixty percent of the membership was female. Their primary presenting complaint was disturbed interpersonal relations. The patients were frequently in crisis, particularly regarding their marital partners, and often tolerated abusive relationships. However, their spouses reportedly refused to seek marital therapy with them. A common theme in the group was the conflict between autonomy and dependency. The topics of separation and loss were frequently discussed. The patients tended to feel helpless, wanted answers from the therapists, bitterly complained, and wept. They described their friends and families as being overwhelmed by their demands and reluctant to give more support. The patients in the group had an average length of stay of two to four months.

Short-Term, Time-Limited, Interpretive Group Psychotherapy (STIG)

The STIG given primary attention in this section was developed for a homogeneous sample of psychiatric outpatients who had suffered person losses. The LTSG patient population described earlier and the STIG patient population shared several characteristics. Both were struggling with issues of separation and loss and tended to develop dependent relationships about which they were in conflict. However, other aspects of the two types of group therapy differed, which resulted in differing selection criteria.

Theoretical Orientation

The theoretical orientation of STIG is psychodynamic. Psychodynamic theory assumes that recurrent, internal conflicts whose components are largely unconscious serve to perpetuate maladaptation. Therefore, the difficulties experienced by STIG loss patients are assumed to be related to the exacerbation of unconscious conflicts, for example, independence versus dependence or privacy versus intimacy. While such conflicts are experienced by everyone and even these patients probably have achieved a partial resolution, it is hypothesized that the debilitating effect of the loss followed a reintensification of the conflicts.

Objectives

The primary objective for STIG loss patients is to explore and negotiate a new resolution to their conflicts. This objective is accomplished by first helping patients solve their presenting problems by achieving insight into the ways their difficulties are related to unresolved intrapsychic conflicts and then initiating a process of working through that continues beyond the treatment sessions.

Therapist Technique

The technical orientation emphasizes an active therapist role in which interpretation and clarification rather than support and direction are emphasized. Relevant here-and-now events in the group, including transference, are highlighted and explored. The therapist interprets themes that emerge in the group as reflecting the concerns of individual members as well as the group as a whole. Patients are encouraged to contribute to the therapeutic process of other patients.

Composition

The relationship between the strategy for group composition and patient selection criteria is particularly salient in the case of STIG. Rather than assuming that general selection criteria must be made progressively restrictive as one moves from long-term to short-term forms of therapy, practitioners of STIG believe that the nature of the patients' problems might compensate for certain "weaknesses" in general qualifications. The composition strategy consists of selecting patients who are homogeneous with respect to a problem that is particularly conducive to work and resolution in brief, time-limited group therapy.

For example, it is assumed that patients experiencing a pathological reaction to a person loss represent a population whose problems are particularly conducive to work and resolution by STIG. As clients confront the inevitable loss of the group, unresolved conflicts and feelings associated with each patient's idiosyncratic loss can be reexperienced and addressed in the here-and-now group situation. Consistent with Mann's (1973) model of time-limited individual therapy, by understanding their reaction to the loss of the group, the patients may begin to work through unresolved conflicts that are associated with their previous losses.

Regarding the types of problem that could be addressed in STIG, Goldberg, Schuyler, Bransfield, and Savino (1983) pointed out that "there seems to be no specific limitation . . . as long as it can be conceptualized as containing conflicts that can be worked with in the time allotted" (p. 417). The authors identified three sources of patient problems: an outpatient psychiatric clinic (e.g., repetitive failures in relationships), a general hospital (e.g., post-mastectomy recovery), and the community (e.g., single parenthood, divorce). In addition to individual adults, STIG has also been successfully conducted with alcoholic couples (Mathiasen & Davenport, 1988) and with early latency-age children (Charach, 1983).

Group Structure

Each loss group is composed of 7 to 10 adult men and women. The group is conducted by either a single therapist or a cotherapy team. The groups meet once weekly for 90-minute sessions. The duration of the groups is limited to 12 sessions, and after the second session the membership is closed.

Preparation

Patients referred to loss groups receive preparation by more than one person (referring source, program interviewer) and in more than one form (verbal, written). Repetitive and varied preparation is much more likely to overcome the anxiety of patients anticipating group therapy. Preparation involves discussing the group's ground rules with the patients. The rules include the importance of commitment and confidentiality and suggestions as to how to comport oneself in the group, for example, to be as honest as possible concerning thoughts and feelings experienced in the group. The screening and preparation interviews are combined for 3 to 5 patients at a time. Each meeting is conducted by the group therapist. The advantages and disadvantages of group screening were described in the first section of this chapter.

Patient Selection Criteria

The following excerpt is from an assessment interview of a patient considered suitable for STIG.

ASSESSOR: I understand that you're thinking about getting into some therapy. Maybe you could elaborate on what's led you to this decision.

DIANE: Well, I've been feeling pretty down for many years, and I can't cope by myself anymore.

A: You say "pretty down." Can you tell me what you've noticed about yourself?

D: I feel depressed, no energy, no interest in anything . . .

A: How long have you been feeling depressed like this?

D: About 15 years, since my mother died.

A: Have you ever been treated for your depression?

D: About a year after her death, I got really depressed—wasn't eating or sleeping. I was on antidepressants for about 9 months. They did help. I'm not as depressed now as I was then. I've just got no passion in my life—no zip.

A: Have you ever tried "talk" therapy?

D: No, I always thought that it was something that would go away with time.

A: Could you put into words what your goals for therapy are?

D: I want to get over feeling depressed. I want to feel better about myself, to feel excited about life again. I have to let my mother go and get on with my life. It's like I died with her, that I literally can't live without her—or maybe I'm afraid I don't deserve to live without her.

A: We have a group that meets once a week for an hour and a half for 12 weeks. It's especially focused on difficulties with loss.

D: How many people?

A: About 7 or 8 people, much like yourself, who have experienced a loss and for some reason just can't get over it. The group is designed to focus on issues dealing with loss.

D: I know there's no magic, but maybe I need to really grieve my mother's death. I have to begin to let go, anyway. How does this group work?

The preceding vignette illustrates many of the selection criteria for STIG. You may have noticed that like our LTSG candidate, Diane has been depressed since the death of her mother 15 years earlier. That similarity raises an important issue regarding selecting patients for STIG: Despite how well patients may be prepared for STIG and how conducive a particular problem may be for work and resolution within STIG, patients differ in suitability. In other words, while certain patients may have problems that are conducive to a short-term group format, the patients may not be suited to work in the dynamically oriented approach.

The variability in suitability is demonstrated in the work of Drob and Bernard (1986). In conducting short-term groups for genital herpes patients, they utilized a psychodynamic approach and a cognitive-behavioral stress management approach. The two approaches have several elements in common. The structure of both types of groups consists of 10 weekly sessions of 85 minutes in duration. Many of the hypothesized curative factors are the same and include relieving isolation, overcoming denial, resolving ethical dilemmas, and exchanging information. The authors reported that the cognitive-behavioral approach is offered to a wide range of patients and is especially useful for relatively fragile individuals. The authors did not specify which patients are offered a psychodynamic approach. They did report that "the success of the psychodynamic group is more variable and is dependent on such factors as . . . the willingness of group members to take interpersonal risks in a group setting" (p. 19).

The general criteria that have been cited in the literature for the briefer forms of dynamically oriented therapy continue to be important—and there is consensus in the literature concerning suitable candidates. Common guidelines outlined by Poey (1985) are presented in Table 1.3. The case of Diane meets Poey's criteria. Diane has struggled with depression since the death of her mother (criterion 1). She sees the connection between her mother's death and her depression as one where she was afraid she did not deserve to live without her (criterion 2). She wants to let her mother go and get on with her life (criterion 3). She is interested in beginning the process (criterion 4) even though she accepts that there are no magic answers (criterion 5). Poey's sixth criterion is not easily identified in a dyadic interview.

TABLE 1.3. Poey's (1985) Patient Selection Criteria for Short-Term Interpretive Group Therapy

- Ability to verbalize a focal complaint
- Significant level of psychological mindedness
- Urge to grow and explore
- Desire to enter a short-term group
- Realistic expectations of the group
- Basic ability to relate to and to be influenced by others

Several criteria could easily be added, for example, a history of previous successful work in a group and an ability to tolerate anxiety in group situations. They are also difficult to assess in the dyadic interview, which underscores the role of a screening group. Criteria that have been emphasized by practitioners of dynamically oriented, short-term individual psychotherapy are also relevant. Sifneos's (1981) recommendations are summarized in Table 1.4. These criteria are, of course, ideals. Strict adherence to all of them would preclude the membership of most patients!

Patient Exclusion Criteria

Given the psychodynamic orientation of STIG, patients who are suicidal, psychotic, severely depressed, or in an acute crisis are excluded. They may need to be hospitalized. If treated on an outpatient basis, they can be seen individually and offered support, problem strategies, or referral to community agencies to help resolve practical problems. Patients experiencing normal mourning are also offered individual supportive sessions or referral to community agencies. There may be a specialty group more appropriate for them, such as a support group for SIDS, AIDS, and so forth. Typically, the suicidal, depressed, and psychotic patients are assessed for psychopharmacological intervention first. When stabilized on medication, they can be reassessed for the group. Those with current substance abuse problems are referred to agencies that specialize in this area of psychopathology.

Patient Population

As part of a recent outcome study of STIG for loss that involved 16 therapy groups, we were able to investigate the characteristics of the patient population (Piper, McCallum, & Azim, 1992). The descriptive information about the patients that follows is based on a sample of 94 patients, the primary sample for the outcome analyses. The sample consisted of 68 women and 26 men. Their average age was 36 years. Over two thirds of the patients did not live with a partner, being either wid-

TABLE 1.4. Sifneos's (1981) Patient Selection Criteria for Short-Term Interpretive Individual Therapy

- Circumscribed chief complaint
- History of meaningful give-and-take relationships
- Flexible interactions with the evaluating interviewer
- Above-average psychological sophistication and intelligence

owed, separated, divorced, or single. Most had at least a high school education; over one quarter had attended or were attending a technical college; almost one third had attended or were attending university. Most of the patients were either employed, responsible for a household, or involved in full-time or part-time studies.

All patients had been assessed as experiencing a pathologic grief reaction following the loss of a person through death, separation/divorce, or both. Since treatment was not crisis intervention, the patients were beyond the initial period of shock and mourning. Nevertheless, depressive symptomatology, social isolation, loneliness, and low self-esteem were common presenting features. In terms of the third edition of the *Diagnostic and Statistical Manual of Mental Disorders* (DSM-III; American Psychiatric Association, 1980) the most common Axis I diagnoses were major depression, adjustment disorder, dysthymia, and anxiety disorder. One sixth also received an Axis II diagnosis, usually dependent personality disorder. Two thirds of the patients had had previous contact with a mental health professional, but few had previously received psychotherapy. About half of the patients reported taking a psychotropic medication, which was almost always an antidepressant.

SPECIAL ASSESSMENT PROCEDURES

As previously mentioned, the research literature offers little guidance in identifying valid selection criteria for patients who will benefit from group treatment. The researcher's challenge is to "empirically [identify] the group relevant behaviors requisite to achieving positive outcomes and then [develop] reliable and predictively valid pretherapy measures of these behaviors" (Woods & Melnick, 1979, p. 162). The incorporation of research instruments into clinical practice was advanced by cognitive-behavorial therapists. They routinely assess patients on dimensions that are relevant for treatment. For example, in the treatment of depression they routinely administer the Beck Depression Inventory. Concepts relevant for dynamically oriented therapy tend to be more difficult to identify and assess, especially by paper-and-pencil measures. To benefit from STIG, the patient must be able to identify the conflictual components of his problems. Toward that end, he or she must be able to quickly and easily form a working relationship with the therapist. We believe that these two abilities reflect the patient dimensions *psychological mindedness* and *quality of object relations*. In this section we describe two research instruments that we have developed to assess these two patient dimensions: the Psychological Mindedness Assessment Procedure (McCallum & Piper,

1990a) and the Quality of Object Relations Scale (Azim, Piper, Segal, Nixon, & Duncan, 1991).

Psychological Mindedness Assessment Procedure (PMAP)

A review of the psychotherapy literature reveals a consensus regarding the relevance of psychological mindedness (PM) for working within all forms of psychodynamically oriented therapy. However, the concept has been afforded various definitions in the literature (Silver, 1983; Bloch, 1979; Tyson & Sandler, 1971). As a consequence, there have been few attempts to operationalize the concept and each has drawn criticism. Self-report questionnaires have tended to incorporate related concepts into the assessment of PM, for example, "effortful cognitive endeavours" (Bagby, Taylor, & Ryan, 1986) and motivation (Conte et al., 1990). While such concepts are important to investigate, "evaluating patients on the psychological mindedness factor involves assessing their suitability only for a specific kind of treatment, not their general motivation for either treatment or change" (Rosenbaum & Horowitz, 1983, p. 352). A second method has been to appraise PM based on general clinical interviews (Rosenbaum & Horowitz, 1983; Piper, Debbane, Bienvenu, & Garant, 1984). Those appraisals of PM tend to be made, however, in conjunction with a number of other variables. Thus, threats to validity have been present, for example, halo effects. Another indirect method has been to derive an appraisal of PM by combining scores from other variables (Horowitz, 1989; Kernberg et al., 1972). That method has the additional problem of defining a psychological concept in terms of other psychological concepts rather than overt, quantifiable behavior.

Given the difficulties inherent in previous attempts to operationalize PM, it is perhaps not surprising that few studies have investigated its relationship with therapy process and outcome. When the relationship has been investigated, the results have been inconclusive. For example, the results of studies by Abramowitz and Abramowitz (1984) and by Piper and colleagues (1984) provide some support for a relationship between psychological mindedness and the outcome of short-term group therapy. However, the results of the Menninger psychotherapy project did not reveal a significant relationship in the case of individual therapy.

In our setting we developed the Psychological Mindedness Assessment Procedure (PMAP) as a videotape measure of PM (McCallum & Piper, 1987). Consistent with previous conceptual definitions, we defined PM as the ability to identify conflictual dynamic components—for example, wishes, anxiety, defenses—and to relate them to a person's difficulties. The videotape presents a simulated patient–therapist interaction.

The interaction begins with an actress/patient describing a recent event in her life to her male therapist. This description includes verbalizations reflecting dynamic components—that is, conflictual wishes and fears, defensive maneuvers, and links between internal and external events (i.e., links between cognition/affects and behavior). The patient's account constitutes the test stimulus for assessing psychological mindedness.

After viewing the patient's account, the tape is stopped and the person being assessed is asked for his/her general impressions of "What seems to be troubling this woman?" The PMAP differentiates nine levels of PM. The criteria for each level reflect basic assumptions of psychodynamic theory. These assumptions include psychic determinism, the unconscious, ambivalence, conflict, and defense mechanisms. The criteria also reflect the ability to identify dynamic (intrapsychic) components and to relate them to a person's difficulty. Scores range from 1 (low) to 9 (high), reflecting the nine levels of PM. To obtain a high score, a person must reflect several of the basic assumptions held by psychodynamic therapists concerning human pathology. The following example illustrates the recognition of a conflict between a wish and a fear that creates difficulties for the person: She wants to reconcile with her ex-husband, but she is also afraid of the hurt she may experience if she gets him back; she is feeling confused.

The video-interview assessment takes only 15 minutes. Its psychometric properties (reliability, validity) were supported in two separate studies (McCallum & Piper, 1990b; Piper, McCallum, & Azim, 1992). The first study involved a nonclincal population of 30 adult volunteers and the second a clinical population of 109 psychiatric outpatients treated with STIG. In the clinical study a strong direct association was found between level of PM and remaining in therapy. In addition, by examining the process of therapy, PM was found to be directly related to working in the groups, not simply to talking. These findings suggest that it may be possible to identify patients who will tend to remain and work in the group prior to the first session. PM was not found to be directly related to outcome, which suggests that there are additional patient and/or process variables mediating outcome.

The PMAP was developed to be an objective and direct measure of psychological mindedness. The standard stimulus of the videotape allows for the utilization of scoring criteria that reflect clearly defined behavioral referents. The advantage of a standard stimulus over appraisals based on clinical interviews is the reduced possibility of the influence on PM rating of other variables, for example, likability. Other advantages of the videotape method are that it seems to be an enjoyable and non-intimidating procedure and time-efficient for both the person being assessed and the assessor.

Quality of Object Relations Scale

The concept of quality of object relations (QOR) has become increasingly significant in the theory and practice of dynamically oriented psychotherapy. Similar to psychological mindedness, the obstacle to empirical research of QOR involves "the difficulty of assessing object relations in a manner consistent with any coherently stated theoretical position and with accepted standards of psychological measurement" (Bell, Billington, & Becker, 1986, p. 733). The obstacle may stem from the fact that object relations are believed to comprise three aspects: external, real relationships with others, internalized relations with others from the past and present (object representations), and internalized object relations that are determinants of one's sense of self (personality). Therefore, conceptual and operational definitions of QOR have differed in the emphasis placed on these three aspects.

When external real relationships with others have been assessed, they have varied greatly and have included the testing interviewer (Kissen, 1986; Shectman & Harty, 1986), parents (Blatt, Wein, Chevron, & Quinlan, 1979), significant others (Blatt & Lerner, 1982; Bell et al., 1986), men and women in general (Kantrowitz, Katz, Paolitto, Sashin, & Solomon, 1987), psychotherapists (Hartley, 1989), and persons discussed in therapy sessions (Hartley, 1989). When QOR has been investigated as a predictor variable in short-term individual therapy, it has been found to be significantly related to outcome (Horowitz, Marmar, Weiss, DeWitt, & Rosenbaum, 1984; Piper, de Carufel, & Szkrumelak, 1985; Piper, Azim, McCallum, & Joyce, 1990). QOR has rarely been investigated with group psychotherapy despite the consensus that interpersonal relationships can be best explored and modified as they are reenacted in the group situation. However, in one study that did utilize it with group psychotherapy, QOR was shown to be significantly related to outcome (de Carufel & Piper, 1988).

We define QOR as a person's tendency to establish certain kinds of relationships with others. It refers to the quality of a person's lifelong pattern of relationships, not just current or recent relationships. Over the past 15 years, we have developed and repeatedly revised a Quality of Object Relations Scale (QORS; Azim et al., 1991). The scale consists of five levels of relationships: mature, triangular, controlling, searching, and primitive (Piper, McCallum, Joyce, & Azim, 1992). At the mature level, the person enjoys equitable relationships characterized by love, tenderness, and concern for objects of both sexes and has a capacity to mourn and ability to tolerate unobtainable relationships. Relationships characterized as triangular involve a tendency to engage in jealous, competitive interactions with one person as if to "obtain" a third person. At the controlling level, the person manifests well-meaning attempts to control another in a relationship; the other tends to be infantilized. The searching level relates to a pattern in which the person appears to "fall in love" repeatedly only to become disenchanted, moving on to the next replacement for the original lost object. At the primitive level, the person reacts to perceived separation or loss of the object, or disapproval of or rejection by the object, with intense anxiety and affect; the person is inordinately dependent on the object for a sense of identity. For each of the five levels the scale presents criteria in four areas (behavioral manifestations, affect regulation, self-esteem regulation, antecedents) and examples of prototypical patients.

QOR is measured by means of a semistructured clinical interview that is typically conducted in two one-hour sessions that are held several days (up to one week) apart. The interviewer attempts to explore the nature of the patient's significant interpersonal relationships throughout his or her lifespan—relationships with parental figures, siblings, friends, sexual partners, health-care professionals, and the interviewer. As the interview proceeds the interviewer tests hypotheses about criteria associated with the different levels of the scale and makes comparisons with the prototypical patients. Eventually the interviewer forms an impression of the patient's overall quality of object relations. After the interview is completed, the interviewer's conception of the contribution of each level to the patient's relationships is rated. The interviewer distributes 100 points among the five levels, depending on the degree to which the patient approaches the prototype at each level. In addition, the interviewer assigns a single numerical value from 1 to 9 that represents the overall quality of object relations.

The psychometric properties of the current QORS have been investigated in two recent clinical studies. Its reliability has been satisfactory. With respect to its predictive validity it has been found to be significantly related to patient and therapist ratings of therapeutic alliance and outcome in short-term individual therapy (Piper et al., 1991) When compared to measures of recent interpersonal functioning, QOR proved to be a superior predictor of therapeutic alliance and outcome. We believe that the predictive power of the QORS is enhanced by the fact that it focuses on the long-term pattern of the patient's relationships and that the interview procedure allows sufficient time to assess the pattern.

PM and QOR as Selection Criteria

Based on our own research findings and the importance attributed to such concepts in the clinical and theoretical literature, we believe that PM and QOR are potentially useful selection criteria for group therapy, particularly if they are used in combination. A patient who scored high on both PM and QOR would probably be more suitable for an interpretive form of therapy such as STIG rather than a supportive form of therapy such as LTSG. Greater ability to identify conflictual components (high PM) would enable the patient to work more effectively with interpretation, and greater ability to establish gratifying give-and-take relationships (high QOR) would enable the patient to tolerate the demands of STIG. There is reason to believe that a patient who scored low on both PM and QOR would be more suitable for LTSG than STIG. Less ability to identify internal conflictual components (low PM) would not be a problem and could actually be an asset in not diverting focus on external contributors to problems. Similarly, a history of nongratifying relationships (low QOR) might make the patient particularly receptive to a supportive, caring therapist. Evidence from the previously cited study by Horowitz, Marmar, Weiss, DeWitt, and Rosenbaum (1984) supports this line of reasoning. The researchers found that "interpretive" actions were effective with patients who were more motivated and who had a higher level of object relations, while "supportive" actions were effective with patients who were less motivated and who had a lower level object relations.

Incorporating these research instruments into clinical practice is an innovative approach to selecting patients for therapy. Given the aforementioned lack of empirical support for traditional assessment procedures and variables, clinicians might well consider such innovative methods of assessment. The PMAP has proven to predict process and outcome in interpretive therapies. It is easily administered, reliably scored, and can easily be included in the practitioners' routine assessment procedures. Although video equipment requires a financial investment, the potential benefits for clinicians and patients are considerable. In that sense the return on the investment may be substantial. At the very least, awareness of the criteria of high psychological mindedness may enable the clinician to listen for confirmation of the criteria while routinely interviewing potential group candidates. In a similar vein, devoting two hours to a careful assessment of a patient's history of object relations may initially seem impractical. However, conventional assessment interviews routinely collect much of the information required for the QOR rating: family and marital history, for example. The QOR criteria can help the clinician organize this information into patterns of interpersonal relationships, a slant particularly relevant for the group therapist.

In summary, the private practitioner need no longer rely merely on clinical folklore and the perpetuation of ineffective assessment strategies. The contemporary clinician can use guidelines and advice that are supported by the research literature.

TRAINING IN PATIENT SELECTION

Learning how to effectively select patients for group therapy, like other complex clinical skills, requires training and experience. Three approaches to training in patient selection are presented in Table 1.5. We prefer a graduated apprenticeship in which the trainee progresses through a series of roles (observer, coassessor, sole assessor) that increase in responsibility and independence. This type of training requires close supervision. Preferably it is part of a program that addresses related clinical tasks such as patient preparation and treatment. Such programs are examples of formal training. They are often part of practicum, internship, or residency training in such disciplines as psychiatry, psychology, and social work or part of the programs of postgraduate training institutes. While participation in a comprehensive training program is ideal, it is frequently not available to practitioners for financial and geographical reasons. Therefore, alternate means of obtaining training and supervision need to be considered.

Less intensive but still formal methods of training can be acquired through such organizations as the American Group Psychotherapy Association. The AGPA offers a part-time training program that can be completed over a period of several years. The program includes didactic instruction at its annual meetings, requirements as a group participant, and requirements as a group therapist, all in the hands of experienced mentors and supervisors. In addition to this program, the annual meetings of such associations routinely offer a variety of other training activities.

TABLE 1.5. Training in Patient Selection

I. Formal training
   • Designated supervisor with extensive expertise
   • Criteria of competence identified
   • Certification of competence awarded
   A. Apprenticeship model
      • Clinical setting with clinical population
      • Supervisor closely monitors clinical work and leads discussion of didactic material
   B. Continuing education model
      • Professional workshops and conferences with nonclinical population
      • Supervisor facilitates didactic discussion and leads experiential process groups
II. Informal training
   • Local settings with clinical population
   • Peer supervision through tapes, clinical notes, or in vivo
   • Expert consultant for inservices
   • Record keeping for continual appraisal of procedures

Informal training in patient selection and related clinical procedures is another alternative. Activities are typically arranged among colleagues in one's local setting and involve various forms of traditional and peer supervision. Clinicians may arrange to alternate responsibilities in assessing patients and observing the procedures either in vivo or through the use of audiovisual media. Patients and procedures can be reviewed and discussed together. In this way one can benefit from the experience and feedback of one's colleagues. Some clinicians find it useful to engage in role-play assessments where one member assumes the role of assessor and another the role of a particular patient, for example, someone who is ambivalent or skeptical about joining a therapy group.

Although these activities are informal—no certificates of completion are awarded—it is crucial that they are well organized and scheduled on a regular basis. Clinicians can share responsibilities in reviewing the literature and identifying new assessment methods (e.g., PMAP, QORS) that can be tried in their local setting. Careful records concerning selection criteria and selection decisions need to be kept, which can be reviewed in light of the eventual group experiences of the patients (e.g., remaining, working, and benefitting). Whenever possible, a clinician who is experienced in the assessment and treatment of group therapy patients should be included, even if that is not possible for each training activity.

CONCLUSION

In this chapter we have considered patient selection criteria for group therapy. While a number of general criteria have been offered by clinicians and researchers over the years, the contemporary trend has been to think in terms of specific selection criteria for particular approaches to group therapy. Selection criteria that discriminate between suitable patients for the two forms of group therapy focused on in this chapter are summarized in Table 1.6.

This matching of selection criteria with particular approaches to group therapy suggests that selection criteria are sensitive to a complex interaction of factors such as the therapist's theoretical orientation and technique and the group's goals, composition, and structure. The profound influence that the therapists' theoretical orientation has on the other factors indicates that it should be clearly defined.

Few, if any, quickly derived criteria from psychological tests or dyadic interviews have emerged for general use. Instead, reviewers have urged investigators to develop measures that reflect what will be expected of the patients in particular groups—for example, relevant interpersonal behavior—even if greater initial assessment time is required. The need to develop

TABLE 1.6. Discriminant Criteria for LTSG and STIG

Criterion	Long-term supportive group therapy	Short-term interpretive group therapy
Psychological mindedness	Demonstrates a tendency toward understanding current difficulties as resulting from external events or other people	Demonstrates a moderate to high ability to appreciate the relationship between intrapsychic conflicts and current difficulties
Quality of object relations	Demonstrate a need for gratification of interpersonal "hunger" and a need for containment of anxiety	Demonstrates an ability to examine relationships in the absence of immediate gratification and an ability to tolerate anxiety
Commitment	Willing and able to attend on an informal basis depending on perceived need as dictated by symptom severity or crisis	Willing and able to attend consistently regardless of fluctuation of perceived need
Goals	To acquire support, feedback, problem-solving strategies, and symptom reduction	To understand the connection between past and present patterns of interactions and difficulties in order to change behavior, affects, and cognitions

theoretically congruent measures has also been emphasized. Some recently developed measures reflect the reviewers' recommendations.

Training in patient selection for group therapy is available as part of formal therapist training programs and can also be organized in local clinical settings. It must be recognized, however, that the acquisition of skill in patient selection for group therapy is a long-term process, whether assisted by formal or informal training methods. Selection errors will inevitably be made. However, if a systematic approach is taken and decisions are routinely reviewed, errors will decrease over time and both clinicians and patients will benefit from the process.

REFERENCES

Abramowitz, S. I., & Abramowitz, C. V. (1974). Psychological mindedness and benefit from insight-oriented group therapy. *Archives of General Psychiatry, 30*, 610–615.

American Psychiatric Association. (1980). *Diagnostic and statistical manual of mental disorders* (3rd ed.). Washington, DC: Author.

Azim, H. F. A., Piper, W. E., Segal, P. M., Nixon, G. W. H., & Duncan, S. (1991). The quality of object relations scale. *Archives of General Psychiatry, 48,* 946-953.

Bagby, R. M., Taylor, G. J., & Ryan, D. (1986). Toronto alexithymia scale: Relationship with personality and psychopathology measures. *Psychotherapy and Psychosomatics, 45,* 207-215.

Bell, M., Billington, R., & Becker, B. (1986). A scale for the assessment of object relations: Reliability, validity, and factorial invariance. *Journal of Clinical Psychology, 42,* 733-741.

Blatt, S. J., & Lerner, H. (1982). Investigations in the psychoanalytic theory of object relations and object representations. In J. Masling (Ed.), *Empirical studies of psychoanalytic theories* (Vol. 1, pp. 189-249). Hillsdale, NJ: Erlbaum.

Blatt, S. J., Wein, S. J., Chevron, E., & Quinlan, D. M. (1979). Parental representations and depression in normal young adults. *Journal of Abnormal Psychology, 88,* 388-397.

Bloch, S. (1979). Assessment of patients for psychotherapy. *British Journal of Psychiatry, 135,* 193-208.

Bond, G. R., & Lieberman, M. A. (1978). Indications for group therapy. In C. Brady & K. Brodie (Eds.), *Controversy in psychiatry* (pp. 679-702). Philadelphia: W. B. Saunders.

Budman, S. H., Clifford, M., Bader, L., & Bader, B. (1981). Experiential pregroup preparation and screening. *Group, 5,* 19-26.

Charach, R. (1983). Brief interpretive group psychotherapy with early latency-age children. *International Journal of Group Psychotherapy, 33,* 349-364.

Conte, H. R., Plutchik, R., Jung, B. B., Picard, S., Karasu, T. B., & Lotterman, A. (1990). Psychological mindedness as a predictor of psychotherapy outcome: A preliminary report. *Comprehensive Psychiatry, 31,* 426-431.

de Carufel, F. L., & Piper, W. E. (1988). Group psychotherapy or individual psychotherapy. Patient characteristics as predictive factors. *International Journal of Group Psychotherapy, 38,* 169-188.

Drob, S., & Bernard, H. S. (1986). Time-limited group treatment of genital herpes patients. *International Journal of Group Psychotherapy, 36,* 133-144.

Friedman, W. H. (1976). Referring patients for group psychotherapy: Some guidelines. *Hospital and Community Psychiatry, 27,* 121-123.

Goldberg, D. A., Schuyler, W. R., Bransfield, D., & Savino, P. (1983). Focal group psychotherapy: A dynamic approach. *International Journal of Group Psychotherapy, 33,* 413-431.

Goldstein, A. P., Heller, K., & Sechrest, L. B. (1966). *Psychotherapy and the psychology of behavior change.* New York: Wiley.

Grotjahn, M. (1972). Learning from dropout patients: A clinical view of patients who discontinued group psychotherapy. *International Journal of Group Psychotherapy, 22,* 306-319.

Grunebaum, H., & Kates, W. (1977). Whom to refer for group psychotherapy. *American Journal of Psychiatry, 134,* 130-133.

Hartley, D. (1989, June). *Developmental level of object representations and psychotherapy outcome.* Paper presented at the 20th Annual Meeting of the Society for Psychotherapy Research, Toronto, Ontario.

Horowitz, L. (1989, June). *People who describe other people clearly are better candidates for brief dynamic psychotherapy*. Paper presented at the 20th Annual Meeting of the Society for Psychotherapy Research, Toronto, Ontario.

Horowitz, M. J., Marmar, C., Weiss, D. S., DeWitt, K. N., & Rosenbaum, R. (1984). Brief psychotherapy of bereavement reactions. *Archives of General Psychiatry, 41*, 438–448.

Kantrowitz, J. L., Katz, A. L., Paolitto, F., Sashin, J., & Solomon, L. (1987). Changes in the level and quality of object relations in psychoanalysis: Follow-up of a longitudinal prospective study. *Journal of the American Psychoanalytic Association, 35*, 23–46.

Kernberg, O., Burstein, E., Coyne, L., Appelbaum, H., Horowitz, L., & Voth, H. (1972). Psychotherapy and psychoanalysis: Final report of the Menninger Foundation's psychotherapy research project. *Bulletin of the Menninger Clinic, 36*, 1–275.

Kissen, M. (1986). *Assessing object relations phenomena*. Madison, CT: International Universities Press.

Klein, R. H. (1983). Some problems of patient referral for outpatient group psychotherapy. *International Journal of Group Psychotherapy, 33*, 229–241.

MacKenzie, K. R. (1990). *Introduction to time-limited group psychotherapy*. Washington, DC: American Psychiatric Press.

Mathiasen, E. H., & Davenport, Y. B. (1988). Reciprocal depression in recovering alcoholic couples: The efficacy of the psychodynamic group treatment. *Group, 12*, 45–55.

Mann, J. (1973). *Time-limited psychotherapy*. Cambridge, MA: Harvard University Press.

McCallum, M., & Piper, W. E. (1987). *Manual for the psychological mindedness assessment procedure*. Unpublished manual.

McCallum, M., & Piper, W. E. (1990a). The psychological mindedness assessment procedure. *Psychological Assessment: A Journal of Consulting and Clinical Psychology, 2*, 412–418.

McCallum, M., & Piper, W. E. (1990b). A controlled study of effectiveness and patient suitability for short-term group psychotherapy. *International Journal of Group Psychotherapy, 40*, 431–452.

Misunis, R. J., Feist, B. J., Thorkelsson, J. G., & McAuley, L. (1990). Outpatient groups for chronic psychiatric patients. *Group, 14*, 111–120.

Mullan, H., & Rosenbaum, M. (1975). The suitability for the group experience. In M. Rosenbaum & H. Mullan (Eds.), *Group psychotherapy and group function* (pp. 415–426). New York: Basic Books.

Piper, W. E., Azim, H. F. A., Joyce, A. S., McCallum, M., Nixon, G. W. H., & Segal, P. S. (1991). Quality of object relations vs. interpersonal functioning as predictors of therapeutic alliance and psychotherapy outcome. *Journal of Nervous and Mental Disease, 179*, 432–438.

Piper, W. E., Azim, H. F. A., McCallum, M., & Joyce, A. S. (1990). Patient suitability and outcome in short-term individual psychotherapy. *Journal of Consulting and Clinical Psychology, 58*, 475–481.

Piper, W. E., de Carufel, F. L., & Szkrumelak, N. (1985). Patient predictors of process and outcome in short-term individual psychotherapy. *Journal of Nervous and Mental Disease, 173,* 726–733.

Piper, W. E., Debbane, E. G., Bienvenu, J. P., & Garant, J. (1982). A study of group pretraining for group psychotherapy. *International Journal of Group Psychotherapy, 32,* 309–325.

Piper, W. E., Debbane, E. G., Bienvenu, J. P., & Garant, J. (1984). A comparative study of four forms of psychotherapy. *Journal of Consulting and Clinical Psychology, 52,* 268–279.

Piper, W. E., & Marrache, M. (1981). Pretraining for group therapy as a method of patient selection. *Small Group Behavior, 12,* 459–475.

Piper, W. E., McCallum, M., & Azim, H. F. A. (1992). *Adaptation to loss through short-term group psychotherapy.* New York: Guilford Press.

Piper, W. E., McCallum, M., Joyce, A. S., & Azim, H. F. A. (1992). *Manual for the quality of object relations scale.* Unpublished manual.

Piper, W. E., & Perrault, E. L. (1989). Pretherapy preparation for group members. *International Journal of Group Psychotherapy, 39,* 17–34.

Poey, K. (1985). Guidelines for the practice of brief, dynamic group therapy. *International Journal of Group Psychotherapy, 35,* 331–354.

Roback, H. B., & Smith, M. (1987). Patient attrition in dynamically oriented treatment groups. *American Journal of Psychiatry, 144,* 426–431.

Rose, S. D. (1990). *Working with adults in groups.* San Francisco: Jossey-Bass.

Rosenbaum, R. L., & Horowitz, M. J. (1983). Motivation for psychotherapy: A factorial and conceptual analysis. *Psychotherapy: Theory, Research, and Practice, 20,* 346–354.

Rosenberg, P. (1984). Support groups: A special therapeutic entity. *Small Group Behavior, 15*(2), 173–186.

Sadock, B. J. (1983). Preparation, selection of patients, and organization of the group. In H. I. Kaplan & B. J. Sadock (Eds.), *Comprehensive group psychotherapy* (2nd ed., pp. 23–32). Baltimore, MD: Williams & Wilkins.

Sampath, H. M., Kingston, E., & Dhindsa, B. (1971). Institutional transference and disengagement. *Canadian Journal of Psychiatry, 16,* 227–232.

Shectman, F., & Harty, M. K. (1986). Treatment implications of object relationships as they unfold during the diagnostic interactions. In M. Kissen (Ed.), *Assessing object relations phenomena* (pp. 279–306). Madison, CT: International Universities Press.

Sifneos, P. E. (1981). Short-term anxiety-provoking psychotherapy: Its history, technique, outcome and instruction. In S. H. Budman (Ed.), *Forms of brief therapy* (pp. 45–81). New York: Guilford Press.

Silver, D. (1983). Psychotherapy of the characterologically difficult patient. *Canadian Journal of Psychiatry, 28,* 513–521.

Tyson, R. L., & Sandler, J. (1971). Problems in the selection of patients for psychoanalysis: Comments on the application of the concepts of "indications," "suitability" and "analyzability." *British Journal of Medical Psychology, 44,* 211–228.

Wallace, E. R. (1983). *Dynamic psychiatry in theory and practice.* Philadelphia: Lea & Febiger.

Woods, M., & Melnick (1979). A review of group therapy selection criteria. *Small Group Behavior, 10,* 155–175.

Yalom, I. D. (1975). *The theory and practice of group psychotherapy* (2nd ed.). New York: Basic Books.

Yalom, I. D. (1985). *The theory and practice of group psychotherapy* (3rd ed.). New York: Basic Books.

Yost, E. R., Beutler, L. E., Corbishley, M. A., & Allender, J. R. (1986). *Group cognitive therapy: A treatment approach for depressed older adults.* New York: Pergamon Press.

• T W O •

THE DEVELOPING STRUCTURE OF THE THERAPY GROUP SYSTEM

K. Roy MacKenzie

One of the basic requirements for conducting group psychotherapy is appreciation of the group as a whole greater than the sum of its individual members. It is this sense of "groupness" that makes group work both more exciting and more complicated than individual therapy. There are several ways of thinking about the group system. Since group phenomena occur in many settings other than formal therapy, some examples from a variety of situations may be helpful. See if you can identify with any of the following situations.

> *Example 1*: You are sitting in a committee meeting and experience initial enthusiasm for the committee's task, only to be surprised at the emergence of bickering, tension, and criticism that seems to have no real basis in what is being discussed. Even the best of colleagues find themselves vigorously arguing about trivial matters. After the air has been cleared, the committee resettles into a constructive approach.

> *Example 2*: You are involved as a member or a fan of basketball, football, or hockey team. You watch an enthusiastic team spirit early in the season degenerate into organizational chaos for a while. Previously well-functioning plays no longer click and the players start bad-mouthing both each other and the coaching staff. Suddenly

something seems to shift and the calibre of team involvement improves.

Example 3: The honeymoon is euphoric, promising a future of untrammeled bliss. Never have two people been so right for each other. Then disaster strikes: an argument, tears, angry words—the first fight. Can the fragile union survive? Finally, reconciliation and renewed commitment occur, along with some sober thoughts about the need to talk about issues and negotiate solutions.

Example 4: You are in a therapy group and feeling great about the level of involvement and cohesion in the air. Then in one session you begin to feel on edge; your toes start to curl up a bit. A negativity is enveloping the group, members snap at each other, and there are veiled asides about what the leaders are doing or not doing. These patterns mount over several sessions, and in one particularly forceful session, you start to wonder if the whole thing is about to fall apart. When you come to the next session, with a lurking sense of dread, you are pleasantly surprised to find that the entire group is busily getting on with active work without a trace of the previous animosity.

One way of understanding each of these examples is in a context of group developmental stages. There are different descriptions of such phenomena, but most of them depict similar patterns. A pragmatic and straightforward schema consists of four stages: engagement stage, differentiation stage, working stage, and termination stage. As you read the following brief synopsis of each, try to picture yourself in a group setting, applying the ideas being presented.

ENGAGEMENT STAGE

It may seem obvious but it bears saying: Group therapy cannot take place without a group. A group, in a serious sense, is not just an accumulation of people. It is an accummulation of people who see themselves as members of a unique assembly. "This is not *any* group, this is *our* group." Without this sense of group identity, the cluster of unrelated persons is not a group. The first task of a new therapy group is to develop this sense of groupness. Fortunately, there are well-developed mechanisms by which this takes place that emerge spontaneously in almost all groups; the therapist usually needs only to reinforce and guide their emergence.

The groundwork for the successful beginning of any group is laid well before the first session. In Chapters 1 and 6, the relationship between member selection and the goals and theoretical orientation of the group is discussed. The basic question to be answered is, How easy will it be for these people to understand each other? By selecting patients who fit common criteria, you build in a degree of homogeneity. This will make it easier for the members to feel more comfortable in the group setting. Common topics of concern will arise at an early point.

It is also useful for the therapist to see each incoming member on at least a couple of occasions before the group begins. This provides an opportunity for the patient to develop a sense of alliance with the leader. This identification provides some security for the new group member and makes it easier to take the risks of getting involved in the group process. If the group is to be led by two therapists, then the interviews should be with both therapists together, if at all possible. Seeing the potential group member individually for a prolonged time, however, runs the risk of establishing an individual bond that may make it difficult for the patient to "give up" the therapist to the group. In some settings it is common for therapy to begin with individual therapy and then shift to group therapy. This is a delicate transition and the groundwork for it needs to be carefully laid.

Priming for Interpersonal Focus

A significant part of the pregroup meetings should focus in some detail on the nature of the patient's interpersonal relationships. Groups are particularly helpful in addressing interpersonal psychopathology. A systematic approach to assessing important intimate relationships is therefore warranted. The following schema has a double purpose: to acquaint you with the patient's principle modes of relating and to get the patient thinking in terms of interpersonal ideas. This portion of the pregroup assessment is therefore directly linked to the early establishment of a working atmosphere in the group. (To begin with, you may want to try to apply each step to your own personal history.)

1. Consider the general emotional climate in your home during your childhood, up to about 10 or 12 years of age. What sorts of images come to mind? Are they primarily positive, negative, or a mixture? What is your role in these memories? Who else is featured in them? How are the situations resolved?
2. Consider your relationship with your mother during this time period. What was the sense of closeness, trust, and reliableness like? How much control did you experience? What incentive did you have to be independent?
3. Consider the same issues in regard to your father.
4. Think of your role between the two of them. Were they more or

less united in their approach to you? Who was closer? Was there a sense of competition? Did you get caught up in issues that really belonged to them?

5. If you have siblings, go through the same examination of each of those relationships.

6. Who were the important people in your extended family? What role did they play in your life? Are there some important role models from your youth that you have not thought about for awhile?

6. How about your peers during elementary school years? Who was your best friend? What was that relationship like? What was your position in the group?

7. Answer the same questions for your teen years.

By now, you should have done a fast survey of formative relationship patterns. Think back again and see if you have omitted any important people, perhaps school teachers, ministers, leaders of youth organizations. Can you summarize what was helpful and constructive about your early years? What was less than desirable or actually harmful?

8. Now make a list of the most important close relationships you have had in each decade of your adult years. How about your first true romance? Any longer-term intimate relationships, even some you might like to forget? Think of the range of close friends. Look over your list and see if it represents a pretty good cross-section of your personal life. Now take one of these relationships from your adult life and consider the following issues:

   a. Overall, how would you describe the way that person behaved toward you? Were they quite loving and approaching, or was there a lot of anger, perhaps even rejection or criticism, involved? Was that person quite independent in your relationship? Even too much so? Or were they overly controlling and involved so that they restricted your freedom?

   b. How would you describe your reaction to that person? Were you accepting and loving, or did you find yourself with negative, angry, protesting feelings towards them, even if you did not express them openly? Were you able to be assertive and independent in the relationship? Or were you submissive or dependent?

   c. Now try out the questions from section a in terms of how you actually behaved towards the other person. Did you have one set of feelings inside and another that you expressed openly

to them? Were the good feelings left unexpressed while critical ones got shown? Or vice versa: Were you pleasant on the
outside but seething inside?

d. Finally apply section b to the other. Think about how you believe the other reacted to you inside. Is there a discrepancy in
what you think was going on inside compared to what the
outside behavior was like?

9. You have now completed an interactional circle for the relationship involving outward action and inside reaction. Can you see
any parallels between this adult relationship and some parts of
the relationships you had with your own family as a child? Are
there vestiges of how you reacted to one of your parents? How
about the way they got along with each other? Feel free to try the
same procedure with any of the others on your list of significant
people.

The system you have just applied is based on the Structural Analysis
of Social Behavior (SASB) developed by Lorna Benjamin (1974). Whether
or not you use a formal questionnaire or just apply the ideas informally,
a rich mine of information about relationships can be tapped. Using a
somewhat structured approach like this encourages the patient to begin
thinking about relationships in a new way and comparing earlier with
later experiences. This is a good way to prepare patients for the group
experience as well as to elicit important historical information that contributes to your understanding of the patient.

Pretherapy Preparation

Think of a group you have recently joined. It need not be a therapy or
training-related group, just a new group of some sort. Think back to the
time just before the group started. Did you want to know something about
the leader and about the way the group would operate? Were you interested in what your role or responsibilities would be in the group? Would
you have to talk about yourself? Would interaction between the group
members be encouraged or would it be largely leader centered? Was it
likely to be a place where you would meet people who might become
friends? These all seem like perfectly reasonable questions to ask and
for which you might expect answers from the leader or sponsoring organization. They are certainly the type of questions patients coming into
group psychotherapy are likely to have on their minds.

Patients should be prepared by a systematic review of what groups
are about and how one can get the most out of the experience. Such "role

induction" procedures have been shown to decrease the number of patients who drop out of a group at an early point. Most premature terminations occur during the first half dozen sessions. After that point, terminations are usually associated with specific events in or out of the group. The main intent of pretherapy preparation is to retain patients in the group until they can experience the pull of group membership that will motivate them to remain.

Some of the topics that are usefully covered in preparation for a psychotherapy group follow (MacKenzie, 1990). One convenient way to cover this material is to give the list to the patient to read at home. It can then be discussed during the final pregroup assessment session or reviewed during the first group session and kept in mind for reinforcement during the first few sessions. This can usually be done in an innocuous way by bridging into it from comments made in the group by members. By putting these principles into words at the beginning of the group, the way is prepared to reintroduce them later in the group when they will have more applied meaning for the members.

1. There is strong clinical research evidence that groups can be helpful.
2. Groups are particularly useful for addressing the interpersonal aspects of difficulties as well as the views one has about oneself.
3. Groups are not a second-rate treatment, results are about the same as with individual therapy.
4. You will not be forced to confess your shortcomings. Groups progress at their own pace and you are in control of what you want to talk about.
5. The more you get involved, the more you will get out of it. Try to be open and honest in what you say, and listen hard to what others are saying.
6. The group can be a "living laboratory" to try out new ways of handling situations, to take some risks.
7. The group experience itself can be an important part of the learning process. What happens between the members and between members and the leader can and should be talked about.
8. The role of the leader is not to supply ready answers to specific problems but to help the group members explore their situations and consider how they might address them.
9. There are only a few formal group rules:

   a. Confidentiality is very important. No identifiable information about other group members should be discussed outside.
   b. Attending sessions regularly and on time is important. The

group is not the same if even one member is missing. Coming late may hold up the group from beginning the session.

c. An initial commitment to a certain number of sessions is helpful. It takes time to get comfortable with the group and dropping out because of first impressions is generally not wise.

d. Do not come to a session while under the influence of alcohol or drugs. You will not be able to get what you deserve from the session and it may throw others off as well.

e. Do not socialize with other group members outside the sessions. The group is a treatment setting, not a replacement for other social activities. The reason for this rule is that when two or more members have a special relationship outside the group, it gets in the way of dealing directly with each other within the group. Secrets may exist and issues may be avoided because of your friendship. If you should have any outside contact with another group member, you are asked to make a commitment to report it to the group at the next session.

The next-to-final pretherapy task is to be certain that the practical details of the group experience are clearly understood. There must be absolute clarity about what day the first session is to be held, exactly where, the starting and ending times, parking arrangements, where to call if a patient has a problem with attending. It is not a bad idea to have all pertinent information typed out and distributed at the last individual session before the group begins. For time-limited groups, this might include the dates of all sessions, especially the final one. Members are apt to be quite anxious about the beginning and lapses of memory are common, so repetition and clarity are important.

All of this talk and the group has not even started! The best way to ensure that the group gets off to a fast-working start is to lay a careful pregroup foundation for each member—to formulate an interpersonal focus with the prospective member and to provide a good introduction to what groups are all about and how a person can get the most out of them.

The First Session

As in all group events, first impressions in a psychotherapy group are strong and color the members' group experience for some time. It is most helpful to plan the initial contact within the "frame" of the group. The idea of therapy taking place within a specific context is fundamental to managing many aspects of the developing group. Behavior within the frame can be addressed much more successfully when the frame is clearly understood and held constant. This is particularly true when treating patients who have histrionic, impulsive "acting out" tendencies.

Both you and the patients are likely to experience some anticipatory arousal before the first session. Careful planning helps to make the anticipation a functional stimulus rather than a liability. Make sure the room is ready with the right number of chairs and a convenient box of tissues. (I have vivid memories of arriving once to begin a new group only to find that the room was locked and I was not sure where to find the key!) My own preference is for good lighting and no central table. Low lighting encourages an atmosphere of reserve and quasisecrecy; tables imply barriers to open communication. Both work against direct open interaction.

There is no clearly right or wrong way to begin a new group. The "atmospheric" principles to keep in mind are tolerance and respect, openness, benign curiosity, and humanness. Gentle but sparing humor will help to decrease tension. Many therapists like to start the first session with as little structure as possible so that members are confronted with the need to initiate the group process right from the beginning. Usually there is a cursory round of introductions. I encourage first names and only a minimum of factual information regarding work, residence, or interests. When the inevitable pause occurs after the introductions, the therapist may quietly suggest that this would be a good opportunity to talk about some of the issues members would like to work on in the group. Here your careful pretherapy preparations will start to pay off.

Almost inevitably, members will begin to identify important areas but with generalizations and in relatively superficial terms. This is to be expected and respected. The important goals of the therapist for the first few sessions are assisting the group to develop effective ways of interacting and reinforcing group norms. The word "reinforcing" is used deliberately because all groups will demonstrate styles of interacting that are both more and less useful. The therapist can be very helpful by "leading from behind" through unobtrusive reinforcement of those aspects that are going to be most beneficial. The idea of the therapist working as an "operant conditioner" molding the group is simple but powerful. For example, a member reveals a piece of emotionally laden information about herself, and another member says she can understand what the first person means, a common occurrence early in a group. The therapist might want to check out with the first speaker what it was like to hear that someone else could appreciate her experience. The therapist might explicitly label the empathic response of the second speaker as the sort of helpful thing that can go on between members. It might be worth inquiring what it was like to take the risk of revealing something pretty important. These interventions would not appear intrusive in the flow of group conversation, but they would underline therapeutic factors such as universality, acceptance, and self-disclosure.

Important early norms include the following. The group is there to work on important goals, not everyday activities or theoretical ideas unless these are directly tied to personal issues needing attention. Members can get the most out of the group by talking to each other and not always through the therapist. The members should have a sense of responsibility for encouraging all members to participate. An attitude of curiosity about what people are saying is very helpful. Statements should be questioned for clarification and more detail.

Despite pretherapy information, it is understandable that new members are not really expecting to look at the process going on in the group room. However, this focus should be established in the first session. Both facts and the emotions connected to the facts are important. This process can be started by gentle suggestions to describe what it has been like to be in the first session. What is it like to hear that others have similar problems? Is there some relief about starting to put important concerns into words? What do the members have to say about the role the therapist played in the group? The overall message is that what is going on in the group right now is a suitable topic for discussion.

Early Group Tasks

The fundamental task in the first few sessions is to develop a strong sense of group cohesion, and this goal must take precedence over any individual treatment. This means that the therapist who is accustomed to doing individual therapy must draw back from the automatic tendency to probe for individual depth. It is more productive to limit interventions to labeling or focusing activities applicable to the whole group. Remarks might touch on themes that have surfaced: "There seems to be a common concern over being isolated from others," or "Making self-assertive statements seems to be troubling many in the group," or "It sounds as if a lot of people in the group see themselves in a very self-critical light." Group theme interventions help the group gain a sense of common purpose and involvement (Piper, McCallum, & Azim, 1992) and, accompanied by the reinforcement of the therapeutic factors in the following list, assist in the development of a cohesive group. The members will attend and report enthusiasm for attending. They will feel involved and attracted to the others. Self-disclosure, trust, and risk-taking will increase and be encouraged.

A cluster of phenomena falling under the heading of "supportive therapeutic factors" emerges automatically during early sessions (Yalom,

1985). The therapist should be familiar with the factors and subtly and consistently reinforce them.

- *Instillation of hope.* The decision to seek therapy and to follow through by starting treatment brings with it a surge of hope that something can be done about a problem. Hearing other members doing the same and feeling some kinship with them and their problems provides a powerful reinforcement of hopefulness.
- *Acceptance.* Being accepted by the therapist in individual therapy is expected. Being accepted in a group is experienced as a status one has personally won. It establishes a sense of belonging and of being accepted that is a powerful antidote to a demoralized state.
- *Universality.* As we have seen, general common themes inevitably arise early in a group. The sense of not being the only one to experience difficulty provides a sense of relief and of being understood.
- *Altruism.* Because of the interactive nature of the group process, members will continually be doing things that are helpful to others. To have this identified provides a strong reinforcement to self-esteem.

These therapeutic experiences almost always occur without much prompting. The therapist is well advised to stay out of the way and let them happen. Quiet underlining of therapeutic factors as they occur will help to make the experiencing of them more explicit for the members. This subtle process of restating, or encouraging, or clarifying what has happened does not sound very exciting, but it provides a major support for the emergence of the group as a group.

There are two dangers in this early group process. The first has to do with the silent member. It is important that everyone participate at least to some extent in early disclosures. The therapist may need to engineer opportunities for encouraging reluctant members. The reason for this is that such members may interpret their lack of participation either as further indication of their personal deficits or as confirmation of their inability to interact with others. They may see it as a reason for other group members to avoid them. Such a situation is ripe for an early drop-out.

The second danger is the exact opposite. It concerns the member who discloses a great deal of painful or highly unusual personal information at an early point. Such members are at risk for leaving the session and thinking that they have again blurted out too much and rendered themselves overly vulnerable in the group. They may fear that the information they did disclose will shock or antagonize the other members. These members are also at high risk for premature termination.

With both of these extremes, the therapist takes the role of rate controller, encouraging the more silent members and dampening the enthusiasm of members in danger of saying too much too soon.

Group Boundaries

So far our discussion of the early group has used rather general terminology to refer to the whole group. A more precise language is provided by general systems theory. One particularly important concept is that of system boundaries. The group can be diagrammed as shown in Figure 2.1, which highlights a number of important boundaries within the group system: external, leadership, subgroup, interpersonal, individual and internal boundaries.

Before reading further, think of a group that you have been in recently and try to picture how each of these boundaries appeared to your eyes. Think of what makes the group special, what makes it different from other situations where you might encounter the same people. What sorts of processes go on between the leader or leaders and the group as a whole? Are there clearly subgroups within the larger group, and if so what is the basis for their existence? Who talks to whom in the group and what is the predominant emotional tone in these exchanges? How self-revealing is each member? What hunches do you have about

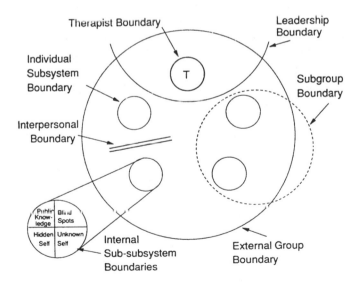

FIGURE 2.1. The group as a system.

what is going on inside each member that motivates that person's participation?

These questions all deal with the boundaries shown in Figure 2.1 and what is going on within, across, or outside them. A boundary can be described as a structural entity. Shutting the door of the group room symbolically closes the external boundary of the group. Membership decisions establish who is inside the external boundary. Simply drawing lines between the various participants based on amount of talk between them will give you a good idea of the communication patterns in the group.

Of even greater interest is the psychological meaning of each boundary. Boundaries are important only when there is a difference in what is found on each side. An analogy would be the difference in ionic concentrations across a cell membrane maintained by the sodium pump. In a practical sense, the boundaries that we deal with in therapy groups are formed by differences of information, of emotional states, of attributed meaning. Boundaries can be thought of as relatively closed, overly open, or with about the right degree of permeability. Try to think of examples in your group where exchanges have been characterized by each of these conditions.

Think again of the group you have been visualizing. Try out each structural boundary and think of the nature of the information that was flowing or not flowing across it. You have just applied a powerful technique for governing a group. Think of the total group interaction going on and try to identify the most important boundary being activated. Then think of how you can "massage" that boundary by being benignly curious about what is happening on each side. By addressing a boundary focus you will be helping the members to make sense of it or to resolve tension around it.

As an example, I recently conducted a training exercise in a teaching hospital by running a group session for patients in a day treatment program that was observed by staff behind a window. It was clear that the group members were not taken with the arrangement and that at the same time they were reluctant to address their concerns because of fear that they would be seen as not performing satisfactorily for the observers and presumably for me. Clearly the important issues had to do with the structure of the situation, not individual pathology nor even group working issues. Picturing Figure 2.1 in my mind, I could see that several boundary issues were being mobilized. First and foremost was the mirror. It formed a boundary between the treatment program as a whole and this particular group. Bearing in mind that a group must be sure of its external boundary before it can begin addressing internal issues, I pushed for a discussion of the mirror. This opened up fantasies concerning who was behind the mirror. It had been explained that only staff members would be present, and this was reinforced by briefly turning on the light in the viewing room so that group members could see that only staff members were there. The boundary was for the moment semipermeable. In addition, the group inside its boundary was beginning to feel its own power and demanding appropriate information. Concern about the mirror rapidly disappeared. To have addressed the underlying issue of trust in the leader would have been premature at this time. The group needs to be more consolidated before it can approach such delicate issues.

The next boundary issue had to do with my role in the group as a relative outsider and addressed one aspect of the leadership boundary. Members introduced a number of complex matters. Did my status as an outside "expert" imply that their regular therapists were inferior? Most of the other groups in the program had cotherapists. Would my presence as a single leader produce a heightened focus on leadership issues? Would this group operate differently than the others? It was already apparent that I said less than the therapists the members were accustomed to. Most of the other therapists in the program were women and the patient population contained a number of women with histories of sexual abuse and of eating disorders. Could gender-related matters be discussed freely in my presence? None of these questions was fully answered immediately. However, the early and direct focus on these boundary issues provided a reassurance that important group structural issues could be addressed openly. Over time these issues were to shift from being important group themes to becoming issues for personal exploration. In the process, the group developed a unique cohesive atmosphere.

DIFFERENTIATION STAGE

Sooner or later, every group experiences the need to address interpersonal differences. The leader is in a position to encourage or dampen this process depending on the type of group being led. If the goals or the capacities of the members make it unlikely that the group will or should advance into more strenuous interpersonal work, then the leader may choose to dampen the emergence of interpersonal conflict. On the other hand, if interpersonal processes are to be the focus, then the leader encourages the group through the engagement stage tasks and into differentiation as briskly as possible. A useful underlying principle is the extent to which the interaction between the group members is expected to be the principal therapeutic agent. In psychoeducational groups, cognitive-behavioral groups, and many support groups, the group is a vehicle for delivering a particular package of theoretical material, but the nature of the member interaction is not the prime focus. In interpersonal/ psychodynamic groups, the experience of the members in their inter-action is considered to be the principle learning vehicle. It may be desir-able to maintain groups in the first category in the engagement stage. Often these groups are quite brief, and too much attention to process might interfere with the other goals. The members of some of these groups have major social skill deficits, suggesting that deeper interaction will take a long time to develop. Generally, intensive psychodynamic time-limited groups that are meeting for a minimum of 12 sessions can be expected to deal with and move through the differentiation stage satis-factorily.

There are some guidelines the leader can use to determine when the group is ready to move into the differentiation stage. Have the goals of the engagement stage been achieved? Is the group cohesive? Have all members taken part in the interaction to a reasonable extent? Has every-one disclosed at least some important personal information? Is every-one committed to group membership? If the answer to all of these ques-tions is positive, then the group is probably ready. It is not uncommon somewhere around the fourth to sixth session for groups to go through a stock-taking procedure, assessing whether it is time to get into more sensitive issues. In that process, a member or two may decide that they have had enough. Most unplanned terminations occur around this time. In one recent group a member who clearly found the interpersonal arena threatening to his cognitive and socially inhibited style put the situation nicely: "I think this train is ready to leave the station, and I'm not sure I want to be on it."

The beginning of the differentiation stage often emerges through discussion of topics dealing with outside dissatisfactions, often with authority figures. Previous therapists, controlling managers, and critical parents begin to appear regularly in the conversation. Often these top-ics have been superficially introduced earlier but the attendant affect now comes to the surface. More interruptions and disagreements develop between the members. The therapist senses that the members are not entirely satisfied with how things are going. Oblique remarks suggest that the group is not getting enough direction. The therapist may be inter-preted as someone outside the group who cannot really appreciate what the members are experiencing.

Perhaps the best clue for the therapist is a nagging worry that this nice working group is no longer comfortable. During a session, the flow of conversation seems erratic and hard to track. The leader may become aware of personal nonverbal responses: muscles tightening, sweating, or a constricted legs-crossed/arms-folded posture. After the session, the therapist may experience an urgent need to discuss the group. It is understandable that the newer therapist might not entirely relish the recognition that the group is advancing into a more confrontational style. But here are some rationalizations to make it more palatable.

If we go back to the schematic of the group in Figure 2.1, the processes of the differentiation stage can be understood on several levels. At the group level, a group that is functioning in engagement processes is well equipped to provide support but poorly equipped to provide challenge and confrontation. Most group members know that this is going to be required. They may remark that there is less urgency about being in the group or that the process is becoming slightly boring: they themselves recognize a need to change the atmosphere.

The individual members also begin to experience the need to have their individuality recognized. The language of the engagement stage is that of commonalities and agreement. Inherent in it is the assumption that "we are all the same." Then it becomes clear that indeed we are not all the same and we might even have quite different viewpoints. The process of moving into the differentiation stage calls for individual voices. An early sign of this shift is often a strong expression of a personal opinion. The leader can facilitate the process by showing interest in how people are seeing things differently or from different perspectives. In short, the leader communicates that it is all right to disagree—indeed it is necessary and helpful.

Within each member, individual development parallel to group development is going on. The majority of people in group psychotherapy have problems related to self-esteem, self-criticism, personal assertion, and the management of anger. They often report a sense of good and bad parts to themselves that seem irreconcilable. Just as the group is beginning to address differences and conflict, so the individual is deepening the level of psychological work by focusing on internal splits. Patients begin to address the anger or negativity that they have seen as destructive or as potentially out of control and the aspects of self about which they harbor shame or self-reproach. As the individual experiences the acceptance and safety of the engagement process, it becomes safer to begin to focus on problematic self-concerns.

The differentiation stage also deals with two complex issues of the group system. One is inevitably the member/leader boundary. The process is characterized by challenges, confrontations, expressions of disappointment or anger and is best understood as a mechanism by which the group can reaffirm its cohesiveness in the context of greater friction.

The group norms are often a focus in the differentiation process. The group challenges the normative expectations that were first laid down by the therapist and reworks them so that they become "their" norms, not the therapist's. The task for the therapist is to act as a wise parent, knowing that "this too shall pass." It is important that the therapist take the issues seriously but not as a personal attack, recognizing that the differentiation process is in the service of group development. The basic guideline is to explore issues without becoming defensive about the process.

Amount of group leadership is another aspect of the member/leader boundary that groups question in the differentiation stage. A common theme is that the therapist is not providing enough. A full exploration of this theme can lead the group to recognize that in psychotherapy the therapeutic change comes from within rather than by fiat from the leader. When the group acknowledges that it has the power to conduct the therapeutic process it is well on the road to the working stage.

The other group system issue that arises in the differentiation stage is more dangerous. The group may displace the negativity onto one member who becomes the scapegoat. The group can then be united in their common "enemy." The assumption seems to be made that if that person were not in the group, all would be tranquil and productive. Of course, the person so designated often asks for the role by being overly blunt and probably too accurate in identifying sensitive themes or issues. Nonetheless, scapegoats often become group casualties, reporting long-standing effects on self-esteem. This is particularly damaging when the therapist sides implicitly or explicitly with the group members in the process. In situations of group conflict, the leader needs to take an impartial stand and, if need be, provide support for the scapegoat. Remember that the potential scapegoat is usually very sensitive to group issues and can provide stimuli for important psychotherapeutic work. A group without members willing to take on this role has trouble addressing more confrontational interactional work. So love your scapegoats and make sensible use of their input!

In one group, a man with a high level of suspiciousness and hypervigilance concerning others' intentions confronted two of the women for "always talking too much." He persisted in this theme for most of the session with a resultant high level of anger and accusations in both directions. The leader could understand the man's point, for the two women did get into lengthy detailed descriptions of outside events on occasion. But his method of presenting it was blatantly provocative and demeaning. The therapist sensed that this was actually the man's way of becoming an involved group member, for he had been somewhat on the periphery of the engagement process and persistently arrived late. So the therapist went along with it, at the same time setting rather firm limits to prevent one or more of the other members from leaving the room.

The therapist anticipated the next session with some misgivings. Astonishingly, this session unfolded with an apology from the man and an appreciation from the women of his sense of vulnerability and need to defend himself. Later, in pretermination review of important group events, this incident was extensively rehashed as a major turning point for the group and for the individuals. The man had learned that he could actually have serious discussions with women rather than treat them casually and dismissively. The women found that they had to address their reluctance to assert their positions and stand up for themselves. The therapist learned a thing or two about tolerating disagreement and sticking with an exploration of the issues aroused.

Up to this point in group therapy, the work centers primarily on group issues and very little on individual pathology. Only after a group successfully traverses the first two stages does it become a vehicle for more intensive exploration of personal and interpersonal issues. The engagement stage prepares the group to work together, and the differentiation stage fosters the ability to be confrontive. These two basic components form the foundation for the development of an effective arena for interpersonal learning. The therapist can promote the success of the first two stages with techniques that deal with group system issues.

Pay Attention to the Appropriate Boundary Issue

In the early group, this means highlighting material that deals with the external boundary. Internal themes of universality and commonalities form the core of this work. Comparison with external situations or previous experiences may help. In the second stage, a focus on interpersonal differences will enhance the work, including the negative affect this generates.

Use Exploratory Techniques

A great deal of effective work can be accomplished by simply being interested in the material and wanting to know more. "Tell us more about that." "I didn't quite understand what you meant by that." "It sounds as if you don't see things the same way John does. Can you explain the difference?" These focusing interventions should be guided by the central task of each stage, as described earlier. By using this technique, the therapist is subtly reinforcing experiences that are most likely to promote the growth of the group. If the group advances, the individual will benefit.

Use Group-Level Interventions

The central task in the early group is to develop the group as a working vehicle. Paying too much attention to individual concerns dilutes this process. The individual is of interest primarily as an involved member of the group. Most interventions therefore should be couched in terms of what is happening in or to the group. A particularly helpful technique is to label common group themes. "It sounds as if everyone is feeling a bit anxious." "I hear you all saying that it felt good to get into the group interaction." "Everyone seems to have a sense that the group is starting to come to grips with important issues." "Dealing with these areas of disagreement seems to put people on edge."

You might want to try more complex group theme interventions. "I get the feeling that everyone would like to say more about their situation but feel a bit anxious about taking a risk." "We've found out that people have brought a lot of common problems to the group, but it's beginning to appear that not everyone sees things the same way. I guess that may make people feel uncomfortable." You will note how these examples have a somewhat interpretive intent but are couched as observations. This helps the group to move toward providing its own interventions without relying on the leader to be the font of all wisdom. Above all, the use of group-level interventions helps the group to consolidate its sense of itself as an entity.

Explore the Experience of Being in the Group

Group psychotherapy takes place through the group process, not through the specific interventions of the leader. Therefore it is helpful to encourage a discussion of what it is like to participate in the group. This approach should be used with every important event in the group. "Well, we've got through our first session. What has it been like for you?" "How was it for you to talk about your grief and even to cry some tears in the session?" "What was it like for the rest of you to hear that?" "We've had some pretty direct discussions here today. I'm wondering how you all feel about dealing with issues that get people sort of irritated."

Follow, Do Not Lead, the Group

All of the phenomena discussed so far in this chapter are almost certain to emerge as a group continues to meet. The skillful leader watches specifically for them and gently underlines or deepens the experience. Such interventions should go almost unnoticed by the members. If the group is getting at its business effectively, then the wise leader will stay out of the way. Remember, you are doing group psychotherapy, not individual treatment. The group experience is the agent of change. The more the group can feel in charge of the process, the more the members can develop a feeling of mastery over themselves and their interpersonal world. The higher the profile of the leader, the lower the profile of the members. A good motto for the therapist is to adopt a position of "masterful inactivity." Your job is to promote helpful events and defuse damaging ones.

Do What Is Necessary to Get the Group through Resistance

The most important guideline for the therapist is to ensure that the group maintains a therapeutic focus. This can be done by monitoring (1) the intactness of the group's frame of experience and (2) the group's firmness of purpose in helping each member to understand important psychological issues. The therapist may need to be active for such purposes at some points—not telling the group what it should be doing but rather guiding the group to find the type of activity that is going to be most helpful. To ignore this responsibility is to lose valuable group time and may result in a group that becomes demoralized because of a sense that nothing seems to be happening.

Resistance to addressing the work task is an inevitable sign that important group issues are being avoided. Resistance is thus an indication that the group is in the right area. In some ways, consistent efforts to clarify the nature of the resistance can be seen as the major task of psychotherapy. An important therapeutic learning task is development of the ability to calmly and directly address evidence of resistance. The therapist best encourages this kind of learning with benign interest in what seems to be happening. A critical approach that implies lack of good will or personal shortcomings will unnecessarily antagonize the membership or shut down the process. Persistently guiding the group to keep at the issues will enable the members to come to grips with the issues. The balance between letting the group take on increasing responsibility for itself and intervening at points of resistance constitutes the art of group psychotherapy.

THE WORKING GROUP

The name "working group" for this stage is really a misnomer. Considerable work has already been done in the group. The engagement process has forced attention on issues of trust, commitment, and self-disclosure. The process of being accepted by the group and to some extent understood despite one's faults has an enormous impact on self-esteem. The experiences of challenging the leader, of confronting others, of dealing with anger have addressed issues surrounding assertiveness, self-efficacy, and toleration of negative affect. All of these issues are central concerns for most patients; the group has certainly been "working"!

The term "working group" is meant to focus on a stage in which the group becomes an interactional field on which individual issues are enacted. The group can now be looked at as a complex system in which the individual's concerns are more specifically addressed. The members of the group have, by this time, become clearly recognizable persons with complex backgrounds. The focus can therefore shift, for both the members and the leader, to individual members and to member–member interaction. Initially this shows in a more introspective group style. Members have a greater interest in understanding more about themselves and others. The context is of course still interactional process, but the content is exploring personal issues, providing the group with a wealth of further information about each member. The atmosphere seems closer to the process of individual therapy, conducted primarily between the members. In most groups, the members show themselves well able to effectively target important issues and to deal with resistance to such exploration.

As this interactional process proceeds, more complex relationship issues between the members emerge, to which the therapist is often in a better position to draw attention than the members. Once again, a largely exploratory style goes a long way. The therapist can be usefully curious about intense reactions or clear distortions of interpersonal issues. By examining these issues under the lens of group discussion, the group explores intrapsychic phenomena. This exploration normally leads with minimal encouragement into further exploration of patterns in earlier relationships, including one's family of origin, although, some groups need modeling from the leader before the members can undertake the work themselves. The leader can help to deepen the group experience by identifying themes common to the group or to several members. Note in the following examples how an interpersonal theme is identified and generalized both within and outside the group. (Note also that these are brief interventions. If you find yourself going on beyond a single sentence, think of how you can abbreviate and focus more succinctly.)

"Your comments about how hard it is to allow yourself to be open with your partner make me wonder if you go through the same experience here, just like Mary describing last week her difficulty in talking about herself here in the group."

"It sounds as though you are very sensitive to anything smacking of control, much like Henry describing how he has to get far away from his mother to feel comfortable. In some ways it must feel that you are controlled to some extent in the group."

"Several members have talked today about their fear and anger at not being taken seriously by their parents. I wonder how that works in the group in regard to your thoughts about how I might react to what you say."

"I guess you're not the only one with those worries."

"The group seems to be addressing really seriously how much responsibility one should have in a relationship, I guess both in here and outside."

The therapist always has the choice of making an intervention that focuses on an individual member, on the interaction between two members, or on the whole group. There is no clear right or wrong way, but it is useful to contemplate the alternatives before actually putting your plan into action. Ask yourself some basic questions.

- Is the person really speaking only from his own past experience without relevance to group connections? In that unlikely event, then an individually focused response would be appropriate. Sometimes an individual response can be helpful in revealing a theme that will eventually be found to have importance within the group.
- Is the person speaking about an issue between him and another group member? Or is he really speaking about his relationship with me? If so, then that specific relationship may need to be the focus.
- To what extent is this person speaking for the group or deflecting or protecting the group from dealing with an important issue? Are there others in the group who have the same issues waiting to be addressed? If you can give a clear "yes" to either of these questions, then a group-level intervention probably would be most effective. With some thought, you can almost always find a reason to say "yes."

Looking at the words of an individual member as a reflection of group-level issues is an important perspective. Most therapists learn first to conduct individual therapy and find it easy to assume that a patient speaks primarily from a self-perspective. But a group enjoys the added dimension of a collective flow of associations to which each member contributes and from which each member receives. In a group that is operating at an advanced working stage, the balance of a member's thoughts and utterances shifts between addressing the group theme of the moment and reflecting the unique perspective of the individual in relation to that theme. If the therapist can accurately tap the group momentum, then interventions have an effect that is larger than interventions directed primarily at the individual. Many experienced group therapists primarily use group-level interventions.

The other side of this issue is that the individual may really be speaking as a representative of the group even though he appears to be expressing personal ideas. The person in a particular role may be well suited to provide a function that the group needs. For example, persons who provide a lot of support and understanding in the group may themselves have a need to see the world in positive terms and to avoid conflict. Such individuals are more likely to be active participants in the group when their own issues are also relevant for the entire group. The therapist may use this understanding of the group process by addressing not only the words of the currently active member but also the entire group. For example, after a period of engagement the group will commonly need to deal with more conflictual matters. At this transition point, some members will be resisting this direction and want the group to retain its warm comfortable atmosphere. Others will spearhead the drive to explore issues more vigorously. Rather than speaking to the individual, the therapist will get more therapeutic mileage by addressing the issues at a group level. For example, "It seems to me that the group is struggling with whether or not it is safe to explore these matters in a searching way that may not feel quite so comfortable. One of you is concerned that things be positive while another would like to challenge things a bit more."

This discussion of levels of group intervention leads to another aspect of the group as a system. One way of describing Figure 2.1 is that it pictures different organizational levels. At the very least, it shows the organization of the whole group, the organization of the relationships of each member with each of the others, and the organization within the individual. These can be thought of as levels in an organizational hierarchy. An intervention at any level in this hierarchy is likely to have repercussions on all the other levels. For example, an intervention such as "The group seems to be struggling with how to reconcile a fear of being rejected by others with a need to talk of important issues" is technically directed at the whole group. At the same time, it may apply quite personally to the individual members—most if not all—who both fear the process of personal exploration and accept the necessity of doing so. A similar statement directed at one member will be heard and perhaps taken to heart by all. Addressing issues of distrust between two members may reveal group-level concerns regarding the leader. If one accepts the validity of this idea of parallel processes at different levels (termed "isomorphy" in the systems literature), then an accurate comment focused on any level should have effects at all levels. There is a strong argument to be made that group-level interventions should be attempted if at all possible, with follow-up to the interpersonal or intrapsychic levels only if indicated.

TERMINATION STAGE

The process of ending therapy mobilizes a number of very important issues associated with loss: grief, anger, rejection, abandonment, not having gotten enough. Many of these issues attack self-esteem or self-confidence. It also implies that the individual must now function alone, with responsibility for self. The process of termination recapitulates many of the central issues dealt with in psychotherapy. Inadequate management of termination issues can leave a bad taste in members' mouths that affects their memories and the effect of the entire therapy experience. Nonetheless, patients and therapists tend to want to avoid this important task.

The first challenge is to recognize and address resistance to termination. In time-limited therapy groups, this is somewhat easier to do since the time of ending is usually established at the beginning of therapy. Nevertheless, a curtain of denial will inevitably cloud members' view of the end. Therapists have a responsibility to make sure that termination themes are introduced and worked on over a number of sessions. To do this, therapists need to overcome their own apprehensions that "not enough has been done" or that they are "abandoning" their patients. To collude in avoiding termination is a significant therapist error of judgment.

Sometimes patients drop out of the group early in order to avoid dealing with separation. "I have never been able to deal with goodbyes," they might say. All the more reason that they should fully experience and talk about the end of the group. In fact it is a good idea to discuss with the group several sessions before the last one the problems associated with leaving the group before the last session. A full discussion of the topic is likely to forestall such actions. A watch must still be kept on members who are the most ill at ease with the idea of ending the group.

The process of dealing with termination will vary in intensity depending on the nature of the whole group experience. For groups that have not emphasized group involvement or that have been conducted over a short period of time, ending will have less impact. For groups that have been together through important personal exploration, the end will be a powerful experience.

The best guide to addressing the key termination issues is to use the model of grief work. This involves grief for the loss and anger at the necessity of it. Echoes of earlier losses are likely to appear, and important reworking of partially delayed grief reactions may occur. It is useful at the final session to have a ritual goodbye from each member to each of the others. This helps to cement the process and puts the termination into finite words. Many group patients have past experiences of losses that make this process particularly profound.

The tasks of termination are conceptually straightforward. The challenge for the therapist is to participate in ensuring that they are addressed without being rendered speechless with emotion.

CONCLUSION

The pregroup preparation establishes the direction the group system will take. A group that is well planned and for which the members are carefully selected and prepared is likely to get off to a good start. The therapist initially must monitor the external boundary issues and then stay out of the way of the group developing a sense of itself. "Staying out of the way" implies that the therapeutic task is executed more by the members than the therapist. However, the therapist plays an important part in reinforcing helpful patterns and in dampening or interrupting harmful processes. This becomes particularly critical as the group begins to address internal differences and conflict. The therapist should always strive to maintain in the group a working atmosphere that provides a corrective experience for the members. The therapist learns to trust the group and let the most therapeutic experiences occur between the members, not between the individual members and the therapist.

It is easy for the therapist to ignore or excuse away threatening disruptions. Tardiness or absences that are accompanied by phone calls and understandable reasons are a sure sign that things are not going well in a group and must be addressed directly at the earliest point. This need not be done in a critical or rule-setting manner. The point is to try to raise and understand the underlying reasons so that they can be laid out as important issues to be resolved. Almost inevitably the behavior represents characteristic patterns of dealing with stress or responsibility. To ignore it is to fail one's duty as a therapist. It has been suggested that the essence of effective therapy is to promptly and thoroughly address any threatened rupture of the therapeutic alliance. Groups provide a wide array of possible ways to do this, certainly more than are usually found in individual therapy.

A similar approach should be taken toward efforts to sabotage constructive work. Talk of outside activities, theorizing about mental illness, and endless descriptions of past events are common ways to avoid talking about the experience of being in the group and of challenging dysfunctional patterns. Such nonproductive talk in groups is best kept to a stringent minimum. Careful preparation and early discussion of major problematic issues can be helpful: Patients straying from their own most important issues can be brought back using their own words. The shifts in focus as the group develops provide some general guidelines for the therapist in judging if the group is progressing satisfactorily.

Finally, a word is in order regarding the role of the therapist. You as the leader have the challenging task of both being in the group and being an observer of the group. On the one hand, your personal reactions to the group process provide valuable clues about what is going on, and modeling empathic understanding may be helpful for the members. On the other hand, moving back out to observe the group permits you to think through the issues being raised and plan intervention strategy. Unless a real crisis has occurred, it is best to wait until you have a handle on the issues before making an intervention. Simple exploratory techniques may be useful to buy time. Once you have a plan of intervention formulated, wait a bit longer. Pick your moment carefully. Try to hang your intervention on the ongoing process of the group so that it appears to be woven into the conversation. Ride the flow of the group rather than trying to direct it. The group will provide the raw material. Your task is to make sure it is successfully processed.

This chapter is entitled "The Developing Structure of the Therapy Group System." In order to lead therapy groups successfully, the therapist must be comfortable with the idea of "groupness." The concept of group developmental stages is one vantage point for understanding the collectivity. Thinking of the role the individual is playing in the group is another. Keep asking the question "Why is this person talking about this theme in this manner to this group now?" Finding answers to this question through the process of group dialogue will drive the experiential learning process that is central to group psychotherapy.

REFERENCES

Benjamin, L. S. (1974). Structural analysis of social behavior. *Psychological Review*, 81, 392–425.

MacKenzie, K. R. (1990). *Introduction to time-limited group psychotherapy*. Washington, DC: American Psychiatric Press.

Piper, W. E., McCallum, M., & Azim, H. F. A. (1993). *Adaptation to loss through short-term group psychotherapy*. New York: Guilford Press.

Yalom, I. D. (1985). *The theory and practice of group psychotherapy* (3rd ed.). New York: Basic Books.

• THREE •

THE THERAPIST'S ROLE IN GROUP TREATMENTS

Robert R. Dies

Beginning group psychotherapists are confronted with an extraordinary challenge when they approach their first group experience: They must lead their initial treatment group without knowing where they are going or how to get there! Unfortunately, no amount of education fully prepares them for the tasks that lie ahead. Novices may spend weeks or even months reading articles and volumes on therapeutic factors and effective leadership, but until they have immersed themselves in the process and lived through their first group experience, they cannot possibly appreciate the meaning of the words they have attempted to absorb. Indeed, the type of comment frequently made by trainees toward the end of an inaugural group experience is "Oh, so that's what Yalom (1985) meant when he described . . ." Even experienced psychotherapists who have just completed their first treatment group are surprised at how much they have learned. Many of the skills they acquired as individual or family therapists do not generalize to the group modality or actually interfere with their capacity to facilitate the group effectively.

There is no shortage of theoretical prescriptions for how to conduct group therapy, but it is difficult for the novice and even the seasoned practitioner to sort through the various models to establish a coherent framework for therapeutic change. Differences exist in the recommended target of interventions, the appropriate leadership style or focus, the nature of therapist verbalizations, structured activities, and the therapeutic factors promoting clinical improvement (R. Dies, 1992b). Although this chapter touches on many of these issues, the goal is not to present a particular conceptual model or to examine critical dimensions that differentiate among theoretical perspectives. Rather, the purpose is much more fundamental: to identify basic skills that beginning group psychotherapists can implement in a range of treatment settings. No assumption is made that the beginning group therapist is an inexperienced clinician. Indeed, many long-time individual therapists may be retooling or expanding their clinical skills by turning to the group modality. Thus, the terms "novice," "trainee," and "beginning group therapist" refer to clinicians who are comparatively inexperienced as group practitioners.

The orientation of this chapter is relatively atheoretical, although my own cognitive-interpersonal biases are undoubtedly evident throughout the discussion (K. Dies & R. Dies, 1993; R. Dies & K. Dies, 1993a). It seems clear that the optimal time to learn group theory is not during the preliminary phases of skill development when so many other nuts-and-bolts issues inevitably confront the new group therapist. Rather, theoretical integration is much more feasible when the clinician has gained sufficient practical experience in a number of different group treatment contexts.

Two other biases affect how the following material is presented. First is the belief that the initial training experience is most efficient when the therapy is time-limited and occurs in a closed group. These features ensure that clinicians unfamiliar with this modality will witness how group systems pass through various phases of evolution, thus facilitating an examination of issues of pregroup preparation (e.g., selection, composition, contracting), early group functioning (e.g., establishing individualized goals, norm building, role clarification), more advanced therapeutic work (e.g., self-disclosure, conflict resolution, working through), and termination (e.g., coping with loss, transfer of learning) (R. Dies, 1993). The closed group setting and abbreviated time frame serve to focus the learning opportunities on these critical issues. ("Short-term" groups generally consist of anywhere from 8 to 25 sessions [R. Dies & K. Dies, 1993a]. Open-ended and long-term groups provide similar challenges, so the types of leadership interventions may not be substantially different, but they have additional complications in greater membership turnover and system-level transitions, e.g., the impact of attrition on other members, role shifts, termination of individual patients [R. Dies, in press].)

The second bias is the notion that the preliminary group experience should be closely monitored by a clinical supervisor who observes the actual treatment experience and delivers feedback to the trainee immediately after the session. Verbal reports of a trainee to a supervisor who has not observed treatment sessions are subject to significant losses of information. Failure to recall or recognize critical group interactions, defensiveness, the loss of nonverbal cues, and similar problems produce serious distortions in the material highlighted within supervision. The supervisor may attempt to recreate the group interventions through focused inquiry or even role-playing, but it is just not the same as observing the group firsthand. Even a review of audiotapes or videotapes leaves much to be desired: Invariably only a small portion of the session is covered as the tape is stopped frequently to discuss group interactions.

"Practice makes perfect" only if learning is accompanied by systematic feedback about performance, based on modeling, selective reinforcement, and cognitive integration through instruction and conceptual refinement. Feedback is most effective when it is delivered immediately and concretely after the group sessions and within the framework of a supportive learning environment. Research on various types of training experiences for group psychotherapists reveals that the skills of the supervisors are pivotal in determining the success of the programs (R. Dies, 1994).

One training format that has been recommended is coleadership by the trainee and an accomplished colleague. This arrangement ensures that each session is carefully monitored by an experienced group therapist, that feedback is immediate and based on a full awareness of what transpired during the session, and that the new group leader has ample opportunities to observe an effective role model. But there are disadvantages as well. Most beginning group leaders simply cannot measure up to the skills of their more practiced colleague. Moreover, the trainee is likely to make unfavorable comparisons, to experience evaluation apprehension, or to worry about how he or she is perceived by group members. The work of the experienced clinician, too, is affected by his or her efforts to integrate the novice into the treatment process; interventions may be delayed while waiting for the trainee to keep pace, and the supervisor may have to take certain "corrective" measures to compensate for less effective efforts on the part of the trainee.

Interestingly, coleadership with a peer seems to substantially reduce these problems while providing other distinct benefits. The sense of "being in the same boat"—sharing treatment tasks with a colleague who is no more experienced than oneself—is generally comforting. The opportunities to be mutually supportive, in terms not just of shared anxieties, fears, and confusion, but of successes as well, typically fosters a genuine camaraderie between the trainees. While they may have conflicts, competition, and confrontations, they can usually work through most of the problems with the assistance of a skilled consultant. The fact that the team is being supervised diffuses some of the anxieties for the individual coleaders.

The foundation for effective coleadership is communication between the two clinicians (R. Dies, 1983b, 1994). An immediate post-session wrap-up is essential, and regular meetings to plan subsequent treatment sessions greatly enhance the quality of the training experience. Some of the advantages and disadvantages of coleadership (Bernard, Drob, & Lifshutz, 1987; Roller & Nelson, 1991) are highlighted in this chapter in our review of basic leadership skills that are useful during the various phases of group development (R. Dies & K. Dies, 1993b).

Unfortunately, many first-time group therapists do not have opportunities to lead a closed, time-limited treatment group, to collaborate with a cotherapist or to receive in vivo supervision of their group interventions. Indeed, many novices complain that ideal training conditions are not feasible within their particular treatment settings and that learning by doing with only a modicum of supervision by an outside consultant is far too often a clinical reality (R. Dies, 1974). Under these unfavorable conditions it is imperative that trainees establish systematic methods to carefully "self-monitor" their treatments (R. Dies, 1980; R. Dies & K. Dies, 1993b) and to vigorously pursue alternative procedures to enhance the quality of their preparation for group leadership. Our hope is that this chapter will contribute to this process of self-improvement.

PREGROUP PREPARATION

The three major issues that clinicians face in setting up a treatment group are selection, composition, and contracting. The bottom line, of course, is establishing the optimal therapeutic fit among the clients, the therapist(s), and the group system. Although these issues are discussed in detail by Piper and McCallum in Chapter 2, a summary will help to establish the framework for the present chapter.

Client selection involves understanding the client's symptoms to ensure that treatment in a group is feasible, gauging motivation for and expectancies about treatment, setting goals, and initiating the therapeutic alliance (R. Dies & K. Dies, 1993a). *Group composition*, on the other hand, highlights such system-level considerations as demographic mix, potential interpersonal harmony, and relative congruence along diagnostic or relationship dimensions (Melnick & Woods, 1976). Unfortunately, efforts to establish guidelines for how to compose groups effectively have not been especially productive (R. Dies, 1993). Consequently, Yalom (1985) argues that "the time and energy spent on delicately casting and balancing a group is not justified given our current state of knowledge; you do better to invest that time and energy in careful selection of patients for group therapy and in pre-therapy preparation" (p. 274).

Pregroup training or *contracting* with group members has multiple purposes. Since many clients have a range of negative expectations regarding group interventions (e.g., fears of attack, embarrassment, emotional contagion, and harmful effects) one goal is to attempt to alleviate the discomfort by emphasizing the safe and supportive nature of the group experience (Vinogradov & Yalom, 1989). Most beginning group therapists have little difficulty empathizing with the negative concerns, given their own apprehensions about group treatment. They too experience a variety of anxieties, insecurities, and doubts about their role (R. Dies, 1980).

A closely related goal is to instill positive expectations regarding group treatment, particularly those associated with self-efficacy (i.e., the belief that the client can adequately engage in the necessary interpersonal behaviors) and therapeutic outcome (Mayerson, 1984). The literature suggests that quelling apprehensions and fears, disabusing clients of misconceptions about their own behaviors and the group's functioning, and establishing optimistic attitudes can significantly influence treatment process and outcome (Beutler, Crago, & Arizmendi, 1986). Moreover, when realistic goals for treatment can be established, the likelihood of clinical improvement is increased (R. Dies & K. Dies, 1993b).

In addition to modifying pretreatment expectations, it is helpful to provide information to clients about role behaviors and group process. Kivlighan and his colleagues (1985), for example, noted the value of helping clients to understand specific skills, such as self-disclosure, interpersonal feedback, anxiety management, and here-and-now interaction. Other clinicians have documented the importance of educating clients about various dimensions of group process (Mayerson, 1984; Yalom 1985). Most important, given the clients' diffuse anxieties about group interventions, is the need to furnish a solid rationale for treatment in the group format. Mayerson, for instance, informs clients that the "group therapy setting is one which provides a special opportunity to interact with others so as to gain insight into one's current interactional patterns and to experiment with new ones" (p. 194).

Pregroup training emphasizes the interpersonal nature of psychopathology, if not in its etiology, at least in terms of its manifestation and resolution (R. Dies, 1993). Also highlighted in pregroup preparation are general ground rules, developmental trends, and therapeutic factors. These pretreatment interventions are designed to form a coherent framework for understanding individual experiences and events in the group context and to minimize the likelihood of premature attrition and therapeutic casualties (R. Dies & Teleska, 1985). Obviously, most beginning group psychotherapists are at a disadvantage during this early period. They have not yet gone through their first group experience, so they can furnish only a general framework based on their readings and prior experiences with other treatment modalities.

EARLY GROUP SESSIONS

Although beginning group therapists are often most anxious during the initial session of treatment, the first meeting usually proves to be one of the easiest to conduct because the basic structure is relatively consistent across treatment settings: Members introduce themselves; explain why they have sought treatment; address how they currently feel about sharing within the group; move to a discussion of confidentiality, outside socializing, and general boundary issues; and perhaps have a second brief opportunity to present personal problems after the basics are addressed.

Based on preliminary readings and discussion with a supervisor, the trainee has already formulated his or her opinions regarding issues of confidentiality, extragroup interaction, and boundary issues, and may have highlighted these in the pregroup discussions about treatment. Nonetheless, it is useful for the clients to share their perspectives on these topics in coming to agreement on guidelines for working together in the group. The therapist guides the interaction, but it is more productive for the members to come to some agreement than for the leader to state the rules of therapy. Throughout the discussion, the therapist fosters client sharing and involvement and attempts to instill a sense of cohesion by underscoring the commonality among group members, creating a safe and supportive group climate, and clarifying the framework of change that was outlined in the pregroup negotiations with group members (R. Dies & K. Dies, 1993a).

Almost invariably members reach consensus on the critical importance of *confidentiality*, but discussion reveals that this issue is not as clear-cut as it seemed at first. Rarely do members agree that discussion of group interactions with significant others (spouses, family members, and close friends) is inappropriate, but they generally express strong reservations regarding being "talked about" to outsiders. Group members understand that sharing their own thoughts, feelings, and experiences about treatment can be very beneficial, but obviously others do not want to be the focus of gossip and wish their identity to be protected. Moreover, members usually agree that any outside conversations about treatment should be kept to a minimum and that members should be open about their occurrence.

The issue of confidentiality leads naturally to the topic of *outside socializing*; members may have opportunities to interact between sessions and thus potentially discuss group events (e.g., in the parking lot after sessions or at social functions; or friendships may form). Since it is virtually impossible to forbid any form of external contact, it is much more reasonable for members to explore the implications of such interactions. Most typically, they come to appreciate that extragroup socializing can undermine their own treatment by placing relationship needs before therapeutic ones, blurring boundary issues and siphoning off important concerns that are best addressed within the group setting where feedback from others may be constructive. Moreover, they learn that outside socializing may adversely influence the treatment of others (e.g., creating secrets that prevent open disclosures, forming cliques that foment group tensions and distrust, and deprive them of opportunities for learning). Thus, members generally agree that between-session socializing should be avoided and that any exchanges should be brought back to the group for open discussion. In essence, they agree with the notion of responsible commitment to the group.

Most other *boundary issues* do not require extensive dialogue. The therapist may simply underscore the importance of arriving on time and regular attendance and prohibitions against smoking and eating during sessions. In some settings an admonition against acts of aggression is essential, but usually the mere mention of this restriction serves only to precipitate unwarranted concerns about the potential dangers of group treatment.

The discussion of confidentiality, outside socializing, and other boundary issues provides clients with an initial sense of security about risk-taking, but such feelings must be confirmed by actual demonstration that the situation is safe for personal disclosure and interpersonal feedback. Following the preliminary discussion of ground rules the content of the first session shifts to more personal sharing among group members, with the therapist searching for material that can be used to illustrate commonalities of problems, conflicts, and life experiences. Obviously, the principal task of the therapist is to begin to mold the collection of strangers into a group of individuals who can relate to each other in a meaningful fashion. This is first accomplished by developing a sense of "universality" (Yalom, 1985) among members about personal experiences that led them to seek treatment and about the feelings of fear, anxiety, and apprehension they share about group treatment.

Maintaining a Positive Orientation

As members reveal their thoughts, feelings, and experiences, the group leader attempts to establish a favorable climate by commenting on perceived similarities, reinforcing efforts by clients to relate to each other constructively, inviting them to share similar experiences, and attempting to indicate how group interaction can ultimately foster change in problematic areas (i.e., instillation of hope). The leader devotes considerable effort to ensuring that all members have the opportunity to contribute to the interaction and to learn that others are genuinely interested in their disclosures. Members are encouraged to discuss their strengths and desirable qualities, not just to focus on symptoms and interpersonal conflicts. The emphasis should be on "softer" affects such as anxiety, fear, guilt, and depression rather than on anger, since the former experiences are more likely to draw people together, the latter to foster tension and alienation. Critical comments about the group are accepted as natural early in the process, with an assurance that negative feelings about the group will change as individuals begin to feel more comfortable with each other. Negative remarks about individuals (rarely made this early in most groups) are pursued to find the possible constructive intention that prompted the reaction or to clarify the impact on each member of the group so that everyone, including the person who offered the critical remark, can become more sensitive to the potential risks of negative exchanges too early in the group's development.

Most beginning group therapists are surprised at how soon the first session ends. Although the need to address basic ground rules and boundary issues precludes significant interaction on personal topics, the clients have taken the initial step toward meaningful involvement in the group. Nevertheless, their commitment remains tentative until they have a better understanding of group treatment and feel more certain that they will be accepted by the other group members. Thus, in subsequent sessions the therapist maintains his or her focus on building a positive group culture. A considerable body of evidence shows that leaders who are viewed by clients as warm, genuine, and empathic, and who demonstrate an active positive involvement in the group process, exert a powerful influence on the establishment of constructive group norms; in contrast, disengaged or, even worse, openly negative and challenging therapists precipitate counterproductive group processes (R. Dies, 1994).

Furthermore, therapists who are open with their group members, especially in terms of their here-and-now feelings and their rationale for therapeutic interventions, are more likely to facilitate the development of mutually affirming relationships within their groups. Through modeling, open therapists promote self-disclosure among group members. Moderation is important, however, since many group members do not expect and may even be intimidated by extreme openness on the part of group leaders. It is also important for the therapist to identify clients who can serve as effective role models and to call upon these members to lead the way toward more open and constructive sharing. The emphasis should be on self-disclosure among members rather than feedback, since mutual sharing will inspire more openness; early feedback tends to be superficial and judgmental and thus creates defensiveness in the group. Extremely intimate disclosures may be interrupted by the therapist with the explanation that such revelations should be saved until a climate of trust has been firmly established within the group. Premature self-disclosure leaves some clients feeling vulnerable, and these individuals may eventually drop out of the group (Roback & Smith, 1987). Early confrontations are diverted with a similar explanation.

The acceptance of feedback is also influenced by the psychological closeness and level of trust established within the group (Kivlighan, 1985). Favorable feedback is generally regarded as more credible, desirable, and powerful than negative feedback. Critical feedback may be viewed as constructive later in the group's development and when positive messages precede more negative comments in the sequence of feedback delivery (R. Dies, 1993). The basic idea is that support should precede confrontation.

The therapist makes early efforts to homogenize the level of involvement among clients in order to prevent maladaptive roles from becoming established over time. For example, silent members generally have an increasingly difficult time getting involved as their nonactive stance within the group solidifies. It is important, too, for other members to share their reactions to the less active participant, since often they assume that this individual is less involved or sitting in judgment. The role of the more monopolistic client is also examined by others to explore how everyone might be contributing to this pattern or to mollify any accumulating anger members are harboring toward their more intrusive peer. A therapist sensitive to maintaining a positive group atmosphere might interrupt a monopolizing group member to reinforce his or her sharing and to invite others to reveal similar feelings or experiences. There will be ample opportunity later in the group's life cycle to confront these deviant roles more directly. The initial goal is to establish the safety of the group environment.

Similarly, whenever other counterproductive processes have gone on too long the therapist invites members to consider what is happening within the group. Thus, question-and-answer and advice-giving formats are greeted with inquiries about the value of this type of sharing, and members are urged to comment on alternatives that might be more helpful, such as mutual disclosure by others. When a particular member has taken a significant risk but is met with silence or a shift in the topic of conversation, the therapist intervenes to process what just happened. Persistent efforts on the part of the clinician to have clients explore group-level issues and share their feelings about how communication may be less than optimal because of these interpersonal problems increase the sensitivity within the group. The goal, obviously, is not to slap the wrists of clients for faulty patterns of interaction but to help them to establish more effective communication. By teaching them early that honest exploration of these difficulties is possible, the therapist is paving the way toward the development of helpful group norms and preparing clients for the more difficult work that lies ahead when more individualized sharing about personal conflicts can be pursued (R. Dies & K. Dies, 1993a). In the early work individual content is not ignored, but the emphasis is clearly on shared concerns about process and commonalities in content to build a sense of group cohesion.

The therapist is in a unique position to call attention to group processes that may impede the development of constructive norms. Thus, Yalom (1985) has noted that "forces prevent members from fully sharing that task with the therapist. One who comments on process sets oneself apart from the other members and is viewed with suspicion as 'not one of us'" (p. 146). The leader's process orientation is important throughout treatment (R. Dies, 1994).

Creating a Coherent Framework for Change

It is clear that during the early sessions, clients do not know how to be "good" group members, so the leader has to guide them through the difficulties of developing helpful norms for group functioning. In the early stages, clients spend too much time talking about outside problems, asking too many questions, offering premature advice, locking into maladaptive group roles, and failing to address group processes that are detrimental (e.g., disjointed sharing, turn-taking, leaving others dangling after a personal revelation).

Unfortunately, these problems can be compounded by a beginning group therapist's limitations. Trainees are often mistake oriented, i.e., fearful of being ineffective or being perceived as inept. They are tentative in offering suggestions and hesitant about following through if group members do not immediately pick up on their comments. They have difficulty tolerating silence, and many of their interventions are "scripted" (adopted from well-rehearsed training role plays or borrowed from readings). Many trainees could also be called narrow-minded and short-sighted. Naturally, lacking an experiential foundation on which to base their interventions, they do not yet have the complex perspective on group process that characterizes the expert (Kivlighan & Quigley, 1991). They are likely to ask too many closed-ended questions, focus too long on less productive group issues or problematic clients, and not be able to anticipate the impact of their comments or to sequence their interventions very skillfully. They miss important opportunities to pick up on feeling words or subtle nuances of group process; even if they do recognize important issues, they are often at a loss as to how to react effectively. Frequently, potentially fruitful issues are prematurely side-tracked by problem-solving efforts or interpretations that discourage further elaboration. These problems often interfere with the ability of trainees to furnish clients with a meaningful rationale for group treatment. Yet, this rationale is essential if therapy is to be effective (R. Dies, 1994).

The task of helping clients to gain a better understanding of group treatment involves a variety of interventions. At a very basic level, group members must learn to become better group members. This is accomplished by pointing out certain process guidelines that will serve to improve the quality of their interactions (Table 3.1). Thus, the therapist counters comments about how "people" feel in a situation with inquiries about how the particular client feels at this moment (the therapist requests "I" statements). The therapist meets "shoulds" with a request for the personal feelings that prompted the imperative. As clients begin to share their reasons for having sought treatment, the therapist encourages more expression of feeling and attempts to engage as many of the others in the interaction as possible; members are asked to reveal similar feelings and experiences, rather than pursuing inquiries with the client who initiated the dialogue (no question-and-answer format). They learn that extensive description about outside events or significant others

TABLE 3.1. Client Goals and Group Guidelines

Client goals for treatment	Group process guidelines
Symptomatic relief	*Procedural guidelines*
Development of social skills	Therapist as gatekeeper
Self-concept restructuring	Boundary issues (e.g., lateness,
Learning problem-solving strategies	attendance)
Behavioral skills practice (e.g.,	Member responsibilities
assertiveness)	Confidentiality
Self-reflection	Outside socializing
Experiencing peer acceptance	Nonviolence
Desensitizing interpersonal anxieties	No smoking, eating, drinking
Modifying dysfunctional thoughts	
Emotional release	*Process guidelines*
Understanding of others' thoughts,	"I" statements
feelings, actions	No "shoulds" or advice giving
Self-awareness enhancement	No question-and-answer format
	Active listening/involvement
	Eye contact
	Openness to risk-taking and attempting new behaviors
	Supportiveness
	Sharing feelings about events within sessions
	No turn-taking format
	Balanced level of participation

is not necessary (group members lose interest, and those situations or people cannot be changed anyway), and that the real focus should be on the personality or experiences of the group member. Thus, story-telling is converted to the sharing of feelings and statements about the self (i.e., how the client felt in that situation, how this represents a recurring conflict, and how such problems affect the client's view of self).

Early in the group's life brief excursions into personal disclosures generate concerns about how others will respond: "Do they think I'm weird?" "What if no one else feels this way?" "Will others accept me or react critically?" The therapist invites members to share how they feel about discussing personal experiences in order to demonstrate similarities in reactions to the process of sharing in the group format and to identify any unverbalized concerns about what is transpiring within the group. Sharing feelings about how it feels to share feelings can facilitate the identification of subtle group processes that inhibit open expression (e.g., seeing others share but receive only questions, token interest, or advice).

Invariably someone will arrive late or miss a session (Table 3.1, Procedural Guidelines), and this presents an opportunity to address a potential group problem. Most clients think about what they have missed but do not appreciate their impact on others. Clients who fail to show up on time or at all may not understand that it was difficult to start the session in their absence, that others wondered about their commitment or whether something happened in the group to precipitate the no show. Open discussion of these issues increases the clients' sensitivity to their impact on others and allows everyone to gain a better understanding of group processes that affect the therapeutic potential of the group.

There is widespread agreement that brief forms of treatment require the establishment of more modest goals, greater attention to task focus, prompt interventions, and more active participation on the part of the clinician (Koss & Butcher, 1986). Thus, in time-limited groups the therapist must help members to clarify their goals in order to foster maximum benefit from therapy. Treatment outcome is improved when goals are well articulated and when group members have a sense that what is happening in the sessions is directly related to their treatment objectives (R. Dies, 1992a, 1994). The therapist facilitates this task orientation by often asking questions like the following: "How does that relate to why you are here?" "Is that something you would like to change about yourself?" "Is what's happening in the group right now helping you make progress on the issues that brought you here?" Too often clients—and beginning group psychotherapists—set goals that are inappropriate for short-term work. Table 3.1 summarizes goals that are manageable in abbreviated treatment settings. Short-term treatment does not allow sufficient time for effective exploration of conflicts that are less accessible to conscious awareness, working through of maladaptive behavioral patterns that are rigidly entrenched, and deep understanding of the pathogenic developmental experiences that predispose clients to personal suffering and interpersonal strife (R. Dies, in press). However, it is possible to gain greater self-understanding and symptomatic relief, increased social skills and peer acceptance, and improved problem-solving strategies.

A significant challenge is translating client complaints into interpersonal concepts. For example, depression is explored for the common social contexts that precipitate the negative affect or dysfunctional thoughts, or in terms of the interpersonal consequences of feeling sad and gloomy (e.g., social withdrawal, irritability, excessive dependency). Virtually every problem can be understood as either being triggered by social events or impacting on the quality of relationships: unassertiveness, social isolation, delusional thinking, low self-esteem. When these interpersonal translations are made, the foundation for group psychotherapy becomes more understandable, especially when it is clear that these outside problems will undoubtedly be replayed in the group setting. As a "social microcosm" (Yalom, 1985) group therapy is likely to approximate the clients' day-to-day reality and to stimulate the very conflicts that prompted them to seek treatment in the first place. Fortunately, the group also has the potential to evoke uniquely powerful processes (e.g., universality, consensual validation, development of socialization skills) to effect changes in the maladaptive patterns.

The therapist helps the clients to convert then-and-there problems into here-and-now issues. Group members who claim that they have trouble trusting people will invariably replicate their wary, cautious stance within the group. The woman who complains that others never seem to understand her feelings can test that assumption in the group and either corroborate or disconfirm that claim. If she is once again misunderstood, she can be led to examine how her communications created that problem. If the others have understood, she can explore the foundation for her faulty assumption. Similarly, the man who seeks treatment for the relief of depression can discuss the interpersonal difficulties that contribute to the sadness, or examine the impact of the dysphoria on how he interacts with others. No doubt events within the group cause him to react with the same type of negative, counterproductive thinking that promotes depression in the outside world and prompts a form of interpersonal reticence in the group that resembles how he behaves in other contexts.

In most instances, the correspondence between inside and outside behaviors is striking, and repeated demonstration of the parallels begins to dramatically illustrate how group treatment can be so powerful. Elsewhere, I have outlined a four-step sequence for making the outside-to-inside translation more effective: personalize, concretize, interpersonalize, and synthesize (K. Dies & R. Dies, 1993). For example, if a client is complaining about a critical parent, it is tempting to ask, "How does that relate to what is going on in the group?" in an effort to make it a here-and-now issue. However, the client's reply is most likely to be "That's why I'm here" or "Well, it really doesn't." It is more efficient to sequence the interventions to get to the point: "What feelings do you have when censured by your parent?" (personalize); "How often does that happen?" and "How do you feel about yourself when you experience those feelings?" (concretize); "How do others in the group feel when this type of circumstance happens to them?" (interpersonalize); "Have you felt this way in the group?" or "How would you feel if that happened in the group?" and "How does that relate to why you are here?" (synthesize).

Many beginning group psychotherapists, as well as their more seasoned colleagues, have difficulty with the more active style required in short-term group treatments. Too often they fear being perceived as pushy or manipulative or rude and so are reluctant to use many direct interventions (R. Dies, 1983b, 1985). However, active structuring, especially during the formative phases of group treatment, is likely to be appreciated by group members, particularly when the focus is clarifying the framework for therapeutic change (R. Dies, 1994). Moreover, when the therapist is perceived as genuine, warm, caring, and willing to be open about therapeutic intentions, members are unlikely to resent the interventions. On the other hand, leaders who are negatively oriented and whose active style comes across as setting limits, laying down rules, managing time, and challenging individuals is likely to be resisted and to create conditions within the group that are counterproductive and potentially harmful (R. Dies, 1983b, 1985, 1994).

Many clinicians who are new to the group treatment modality have difficulty balancing their activity level in the group, and this results from a number of common problems. First and foremost, they fail to "think group" and attempt to do individual therapy in the group setting (R. Dies, 1980). For example, as clients reveal personal problems, the therapist asks for further elaboration, rather than inviting others to become involved in a sharing process. Not surprisingly, this problem occurs more with clinicians who have had extensive one-on-one therapy experience before they enter the group. On the other hand, less practiced clinicians are also likely to ask closed-ended questions that force a follow-up probe: "Does that happen very often?" or "Do others feel that way?" rather than "Can you tell us more about that?" They have difficulty with silence and jump in too quickly. They remain focused on the individual talking (eye contact) rather than nonverbally directing attention to others who might contribute. They ask too many questions rather than reflecting feelings in their interventions. As the next individual talks they feel obliged to comment rather than waiting for a group member to contribute. They are not efficient in directing clients to assume more responsibility, which forces the leader to remain active in maintaining the task orientation; the focus is given to the individual (e.g., "Can you tell us how that makes you feel?") rather than directed to the group (e.g., "That sounds like an experience many of you can relate to. Can we spend some time sharing our experiences and feelings about that?"). And they do not directly tell group members that they would like them to interact spontaneously rather than waiting for the therapist to assume responsibility. These tendencies encourage clients to assume a relatively passive stance within the group.

If cotherapists are leading the group, the problems of balancing the level of therapist activity may be even more pronounced. Many inexperienced group psychotherapists assume that the contributions of the leaders to the group process should be comparable, and generally that translates into an equal amount of verbal input per session. Thus, if either one feels that he or she has not been sufficiently active, a number of concerns may arise: "Am I carrying my fair share?" "Will the clients, supervisor, or my cotherapist judge me to be less effective because I am contributing less?" Their preoccupation is with quantity rather than quality of participation, and they have not yet developed a broad perspective that allows for variation across sessions regarding respective levels of contribution. The cotherapists have not yet developed a sense of how to communicate with each other during the sessions, either verbally or nonverbally (indeed, they rarely interact), and when one leader offers a comment to the group, it is often promptly followed by an intervention by the other. This one-two punch makes it difficult for clients to interact spontaneously, because they come to expect this pattern of leader intervention.

In time, insecurities about leadership subside, and issues of competition become less salient. The regular cotherapist meetings between treatment sessions and consultations with the supervisor facilitate an examination of these interpersonal dynamics. The trainees learn that compatibility despite dissimilarity appears to be the key factor in the effectiveness of a cotherapy team (R. Dies, 1983b).

TRANSITION PERIOD

In the early group sessions, most clients come to realize that treatment requires a great deal of work. Many, despite their genuine desire for symptomatic relief, prefer to have the therapist guide the process and are reluctant to assume responsibility for candid self-disclosure and exposure to critical examination by others. Indeed, those who have problems with intimacy, interpersonal trust, and confrontation and/or those who have failed to experience much support within the group may decide to drop out at this point (Roback & Smith, 1987). For others, the interpersonal compromises required to conform to group norms may be too demanding, and they begin to resist the various requests for openness and risk-taking.

Many models of group development have described this as a period of rebellion and struggle for differentiation (e.g., MacKenzie, 1987), emphasizing issues of control, dominance, and anger as members wrestle with a variety of questions about group treatment: "Can I really risk being myself in here?" "Will others genuinely honor the confidentiality guideline?" "How much are we really alike?" "Can I still be an individual in here?" "How safe is it to disagree?" "Will the therapist be able to handle conflict or will it get out of hand?" It is important for the group therapist to confront these potential group obstacles as they arise (K. Dies & R. Dies, 1993) but perhaps even more important to anticipate their occurrence as natural in the evolution of the group system. Often particular group members are outspoken about their doubts or discontents and assume a relatively critical or resistive stance. Clients who adopt these "cautionary" and "divergent" roles (Livesley & MacKenzie, 1983) provide valuable opportunities to address underlying tensions that can be worked through for the group's benefit (e.g., Bahrey, McCallum, & Piper, 1991; R. Dies & Teleska, 1985).

Yet many inexperienced group therapists are intimidated by these challenges and feel that members are questioning their ability to lead the group effectively. In response, they either increase their activity in order to comply with the members' requests for more structure, or they attempt to shift the focus to more positive topics, thereby stifling honest expression about difficult issues. Such countertransferential responses are less likely when it is understood that "attacks" on the leader are motivated by the desire to make the group environment a safer place for therapeutic work where members can maintain a sense of individuality within the group system. MacKenzie (1990) notes that the basic task of the therapist at this stage of client differentiation is to help members tolerate interpersonal differences and learn how to resolve conflicts constructively, thereby contributing to the normative development of the group. Thus, it is useful to support the clients' willingness to confront the leader, to have them explore the feelings behind their challenges, and to help them understand how they can work with the therapist to create a more effective climate for individual risk-taking.

Their questions and challenges should be accepted as both important and natural.

Unfortunately, therapists too often interpret these behaviors as either a form of individual resistance or group-level flight from therapeutic work. Although it is certainly true that clients are both consciously and unconsciously reluctant to expose their vulnerabilities and that they may even collude in resistance, it is also likely that many obstacles to group process are simply due to the clients' uncertainty about how to proceed effectively. Thus, rather than interpreting the resistance, it is often more valuable for the therapist to translate group conflict and resistance as natural, that is, to normalize it, and then attempt to work with clients to reduce the need for defensiveness. Generally, reluctance to engage in meaningful therapeutic work derives from two major sources, fear of personal vulnerability and ambiguity about the nature of the task. The therapist's efforts to foster interpersonal support and cohesion and to clarify the framework for change both serve to reduce the need for personal guardedness.

Most clients do not enter therapy with a clear understanding of how group treatments promote change. Their ideas about how individuals overcome personal dilemmas and interpersonal conflicts are frequently based on popularized accounts of individual therapy involving intensive uncovering of childhood traumas until flashes of insight are achieved and pent-up emotions are released, thereby effecting therapeutic "cure" (R. Dies, in press). From the clients' point of view, the goal is to discuss personal problems in outside relationships, many of which derive from earlier experiences (the so-called skeletons in the closet) and so must be reviewed in historical perspective. Moreover, clients assume that it is primarily the group leader's responsibility to promote therapeutic change; they view other group members as secondary and their role as confined to asking questions, giving advice, and sharing similar experiences. They, in turn, will have their opportunities for therapeutic change as the focus rotates around the membership. Often, the expectation is that with sufficient probing and self-examination, insight will be gained and emotional catharsis will then be possible. The patients' model of therapeutic change is outlined in the first column of Table 3.2.

It is up to the therapist to illustrate a model of change that is more effective (column 2). Thus, while some discussion of outside and even historically based problems is inevitable, the vital importance of interpersonal translations, here-and-now activation, and the "group as the agent of change" must be spotlighted. It is the process of mutual exploration and sharing, not turn-taking, advising (psychologizing), and question-and-answering, that facilitates therapeutic understanding and improvement. The complementary processes of self-disclosure and interpersonal feedback are pivotal in the pursuit of self-awareness, cognitive restruc-

TABLE 3.2. Change in Group Treatments

Patients' view	Therapists' view

Share an "outside" problem
  Personal/individual
  Historical (skeletons in closet)
	Manifest problems in the group
	  Interpersonal/interactional
	  Here-and-now activation

Therapist as healer	Group as healer

Question-and-answer format
  Advice
  Psychological interpretation
  Turn-taking
	Mutual exploration
	  Self-disclosure
	  Interpersonal feedback
	  Behavioral practice

Acquisition of insight ("aha")	Increased understanding
Cathartic relief (personal emotional release)	Corrective emotional experience (interpersonal encounter)
Symptomatic cure	Improved coping and symptomatic relief

turing, insight into others, and behavioral change. Members (and beginning group psychotherapists) require some time to understand how change occurs through intensive group interaction, but it is imperative that the general framework is established during the transition period as the group moves toward the individualized work that is the focus in the working phase of group treatment.

Strong affective expression (catharsis) may indeed lead to a sense of release, especially if the client is met by the others with genuine support, efforts to understand, and sharing. The care and acceptance of comembers may foster greater self-acceptance, and "putting feelings on the table" may permit more objective exploration and sorting through confusion, which in turn can result in increased self-understanding. Clients can be encouraged to explore the intensity of their feelings, to place their reactions in a more realistic perspective, and to weigh the pros and cons of holding onto such feelings in light of the changes that have occurred in their lives over the years. Clients might also explore other courses of action they might take in situations before their feelings escalate disproportionately: Instead of permitting anger to mount to a sense of rage, they might learn to respond promptly when significant others trigger their dissatisfaction.

Similarly, the group can be used to allow clients to evaluate their interpersonal assumptions. Thus, group members might first share what they want most from others in their lives (e.g., respect, affection, recognition) or how they wish to be viewed by others as people (e.g., friendly, competent, sincere). They can describe how they attempt to generate these reactions and then consider how that style has been evident in the group. The client can be asked, "How have others responded?" "Have you indeed been judged as friendly or sincere?" For example, a female client who has worked hard to show genuine interest in others and thus gain their respect and admiration may discover that fellow group members have been "turned off" by what they see as phony concern. The outcome she has so diligently pursued has eluded her, as it probably does in many outside relationships and will continue to do so until she realizes how her own actions undermine the goals she strives so earnestly to achieve. Constructive feedback from comembers may allow her to discover new ways to express herself and thereby gain interpersonal acceptance.

These types of learning processes seem straightforward, but it is difficult to convey their full meaning until group members (and, once again, beginning group therapists) have witnessed how change can occur. The therapist must attend to small increments in the clients' progress toward therapeutic goals, reinforce improved social skills within treatment, and create the expectancy of more substantial gains if group members continue to take risks in exploring their interpersonal problems: "I know that we've only seen the tip of the iceberg on this issue . . . but as each of you shares what it's really like to be you, with all your insecurities, doubts, and disappointments, and as you reveal what you want to change most about yourself as a person, we can do some very meaningful work together in the group."

The therapist must increasingly encourage members to assume responsibility for therapeutic work. Indeed, many interventions should be questions designed to encourage members to tune in to subtle group processes and become more actively engaged: "How do you feel about what's occurring?" "What do you think would have happened had you said that?" "Why don't we go around and share how we react to that?" Clarifications, interpretations, and disclosures are followed by efforts to involve clients in revealing their own feelings and reactions. An explicit message is that members have the responsibility for what transpires during treatment. If they are not pleased with how the sessions are unfolding or with their own progress, they have the opportunity to redirect the focus. The therapist may ask, "What can you do to improve what happens during the sessions?" or comment, "The group is yours to make of it what you will" or, somewhat more forcefully, "You will get out of this experience only what you put into it." Sensitivity to clients' reservations is essential, yet clients also need to be nudged to maximize their therapeutic gains, particularly in short-term treatments. The basic idea is to create a "leaderful group" (Yalom, 1985); rather than leaving the leading to one or two designated therapists, it is much more valuable to think that each client serves as a therapist for the others, not as an expert in psychopathology or group dynamics, but as someone who, along with the others, can provide emotional support and consensual validation of interpersonal styles (R. Dies & K. Dies, 1993a).

Clients are less threatened about taking personal risks when they know that others are likely to join them at similar levels of disclosure. It is useful, therefore, for the therapist to activate a search for common themes so that several individuals can explore personal material concurrently. Although the specific reasons that bring clients to therapy may differ widely, the emotional undercurrents and the doubts about ability to cope effectively are common. Thus, the goal is to search for the affect and/or the feelings about self behind the events that create the problems. A person who consistently retreats in the face of conflict and another who repeatedly becomes embroiled in confrontational exchanges may seem quite different at first glance. Yet they may both share the same kinds of anxiety and resentment as well as profound problems with self-esteem. So, too, might the client who is having recurring bouts of depression and the one who has a history of alcohol abuse. While the symptoms of the four people (withdrawal, argumentativeness, depression, and alcoholism) are quite different, these clients can relate with each other on the core issues of painful affect and/or self-dissatisfaction, as well as the desire to change self-defeating patterns.

Although leaders should intervene to involve as many clients in the discussion as possible, it is unlikely that every member of the group will become involved in each topic that is explored. Nevertheless, as the focus of conversation changes it will be valuable to find a way to connect those who were previously less active. Over time, these "shifting subgroups" will involve all of the members (K. Dies & R. Dies, 1993). While considerable observational learning occurs within group treatments, the available evidence suggests that clients who risk revealing themselves to others and those who immediately and consistently invest in the give and take of both positive and negative feedback are the ones who ultimately show the most therapeutic benefit (K. Dies & R. Dies, 1993; Tschuschke & Dies, 1994).

Two additional issues may be important to mention briefly before moving on to the working phase of group treatment. The first of these is the issue of confrontation. The beginning group leaders' insecurities about performance, concerns about being disliked, fears of retaliation, and other uncomfortable feelings make it difficult for them to confront more outspoken or resistive clients. Yet clients can be confronted directly without any untoward effects. In fact, clients will generally acknowledge that confrontation by the therapist is one of the most effective forms of intervention (R. Dies, 1994), especially when the quality of the client--therapist relationship and the overall group climate are supportive.

Thus, confrontation does not have to be expressed by the therapist as "giving them hell" or experienced as an assault by group members if several guidelines are followed.

1. *Therapists should avoid interpreting or labeling the behavior and attempt to remain as descriptive as possible* (Egan, 1986). Noting the behaviors, pointing out the inconsistencies, and describing the consequences will generally be more effective than saying, "Your insensitive interruptions . . . ," "Your need to be most important . . . ," "You *always* try to prove . . . ," or other provocative remarks; in short, clients should not end up feeling put down.

2. *Confrontations should come from a position of therapeutic neutrality.* While there are certainly occasions when honest expressions of anger, hurt, of other feelings are appropriate, it is generally best to be perceived as being objective. In this regard, it is often useful to rely on other members to assist in confronting a particular client since (it is likely that others are responding to the difficult client in a similar fashion). However, the therapist should be careful not to act out through the other clients to silence an offensive member, nor should the particular member feel ganged up on by the group members.

3. *The self-defeating nature of the problematic behavior should be sensitively highlighted.* Acknowledging confusion or "playing dumb" may be helpful: "I'm confused right now. You are coming here for help, but it seems to me that you are working really hard to avoid getting it. Can you help us understand what is going on?" It is also important to realize that some of the offending behaviors are not group-specific resistance but generalized maladaptive interpersonal styles. Therefore, the confrontation should be designed not to twist the arms of clients into changing but to invite them to consider alternative ways of interacting. For example, the silent member can be persistently encouraged to become involved and even given the therapeutic assignment of talking during sessions to see how trying on new behaviors creates opportunities for learning.

4. *Therapists can share and invite other clients to reveal their feelings about the specific client's problematic behaviors.* "When you sit in silence, I feel that you don't care about what I have to say." "Each time you interrupt me, I feel frustrated, like you aren't really listening to me." Such sharing is a first step toward exploration and increased understanding.

The issue of therapist self-disclosure is a controversial one (R. Dies, 1977, 1983b, 1994), but most trainees soon discover that sharing their own feelings during treatment can be highly effective: It can encourage group members to become more open, it tends to demystify leadership, which in turn contributes to the meaningful and supportive climate that is so important in group treatment, and it allows therapists to deal with group process issues in a much more direct and forthright fashion. Too often, beginning group psychotherapists suppress personal feelings that might better be verbalized. Indeed, one of my most frequent inquiries during supervision is "What would have happened had you said that?" in an effort to encourage trainees to feel free to express themselves. Unfortunately, novices have heard that therapist self-disclosure is inappropriate, and many attempt to hide behind their professional role or fear that their feelings are not shared by others within the group.

Once again, a few guidelines may be useful.

1. *Extensive and intimate sharing about outside topics by the therapist is inappropriate, but acknowledgement of normal human reactions is quite acceptable* (e.g., grief over the loss of a loved one, disappointment in being spurned by a friend, frustration in the face of failure). Similarly, open sharing of feelings about events within treatment can be productive. After all, many of these reactions, too, are quite normal (e.g., anxiety during a first session, feeling defensive after being strongly criticized, embarrassment after a foolish comment). There is nothing wrong with being normal.

2. *The therapist can use his or her own feelings as a barometer of what is going on during treatment.* Feeling confused, bored by the discussion, or pushed away by a client may be an important signal of what is going on during treatment. It is not always necessary to share what the therapist is experiencing, but it may be useful to call a simple timeout to explore how others are feeling. Even if the therapist's feelings are off base, the intervention may be helpful to focus interactions more sharply. Beginning therapists also worry that they have to know why they have certain feelings and to know how to go somewhere with the discussion, but neither is true. Working together with clients to find solutions during the group's evolution is a major part of the learning process during treatment.

3. *Honest expression of feelings by the therapist can be very effective.* "I'm feeling confused right now and not sure where we are going with this discussion. Is anyone else feeling that way?" "I'm feeling concerned for Peggy right now. She just took a big risk, and no one responded."

4. *It is useful for therapists to verbalize their dilemmas.* "I'm feeling on the spot right now because many of you want me to provide more structure, but if I do that, we might not explore why that is important right now." "Frank, I felt your sadness and wanted to reach out to you, but I wasn't sure how you would respond."

5. *It is helpful for the therapist to be open about therapeutic rationale.*
"John, the reason I'm cutting you off right now is that I want to make
sure that Mary feels okay before we move on; we'll come right back to
you." "I think it's too early in the group to get into strong confrontation.
I think we need to build some trust with each other first."

The presence of a cotherapist during the transition period of group
development is extremely helpful. It is far too easy for less experienced
group psychotherapists to become "hung up on" the members' complaints about leadership. When there are two group leaders, even if both
are trainees, such countertransference reactions are less likely to occur.
By now, the cotherapists have learned how to balance some of their sty-
listic differences and worked through some of their concerns about competition. Nevertheless, they still often find themselves working at cross-
purposes without an effective means of dealing with the problem during
the treatment sessions. It is helpful for them to develop ways to check in
with each other during group interactions: "Mary, I'm still responding
to what happened a few minutes ago. Is it okay if we go back to that before
we move on?" or "Pat, can we call a timeout for a second and try to clarify
what's going on?"

Of course, the coleaders should have a clear understanding about
how to relate to each other during the treatment sessions. Generally, it
is easy for therapists to agree on the acceptability of questioning each
other about therapeutic rationale, but they must also learn that sometimes it is simply best to trust where their partner is going with a particular issue to see how it plays out. Given the enormous complexity of group
process, the options for how to intervene at a given moment are diverse;
there is no one right way to be a perfect therapist. While differences of
opinion between group therapists on how to proceed can often be worked
through effectively during the sessions, open conflict and tension can
be detrimental (R. Dies, 1983b; R. Dies, Mallet, & Johnson, 1979).

WORKING SESSIONS

Considerable work has already occurred by the time the group moves to
the stage of development that is typically called the working group (e.g.,
MacKenzie, 1990 and Chapter 2, this volume). Nothing dramatically new
begins to happen, but there is a gradual shift in the therapist's focus from
group-centered and process-related interventions to more individual,
content-oriented techniques. The supportive and coherent group system
that has evolved now provides a foundation of intermember bonding that
will allow clients to address the specific personal distress and maladap-

tive interpersonal patterns that brought them to treatment. Early but nonspecific therapeutic factors such as hope, altruism, universality, and cohesiveness have paved the way for such psychological work factors as catharsis, interpersonal learning, and insight (R. Dies, 1993; MacKenzie, 1987). The therapist increases the intimacy of client self-disclosures, enriches the value of interpersonal feedback, and shapes the types of interactions that will promote behavioral practice, cognitive restructuring, and emotional release.

The trainees' confidence has increased considerably by this time, and they are likely to have developed a greater understanding of group process and to be more comfortable with both open and active interventions. Nevertheless, a new set of challenges awaits trainees as they attempt to exploit the therapeutic potential of the group system. They have not yet developed their "third ear" and still miss subtle opportunities for timely interventions, and although they understand that they must plunge the group into more significant affect and personal exploration, their leadership skills are not sufficiently refined to allow for this more sophisticated work. Thus, they are inclined to play "head-shrinking" games by offering premature interpretations, problem-solving advice, or such pat phrases as "What I hear you saying is . . . ," "What does the group feel about that?" or "How does that make you feel?" (repetitively and with little variation). They follow guidelines but still genuinely fail to completely understand "what we do when we get there." That is, they prompt affective expression and foster intimate revelations but then do not know how to harness the therapeutic power of intensive interpersonal exchange. Like their clients, they struggle to find the most effective means to use the group system to optimize clinical gain.

Clearly, change in group treatments involves no universal mechanisms but rather a range of factors that operate across clinical settings, diagnostic compositions, and forms of group therapy (R. Dies, 1993). Different clients may benefit from various therapeutic ingredients within the same group (Lieberman, 1989), and the availability of multiple sources of learning within sessions may be more important than any limited set of common dimensions (Lieberman, 1983). There appears to be a confluence of nonspecific factors (e.g., cohesiveness) working in concert with cognitive, affective, and behavioral ingredients (self-understanding, catharsis, and interpersonal learning and social skills acquisition, respectively) to facilitate therapeutic gain (R. Dies, 1991). The therapist intervenes at each of these levels in order to optimize the group's potential for each member.

Treatment will be most effective if clients are able to identify a clear set of personal priorities. When they enter group treatment most clients establish target goals that are rather vague and ill-defined: "To learn how to express my feelings," "To learn how to trust other people more," "To understand how to control my panic attacks," and so forth. During the earlier sessions, efforts to clarify these goals are partially successful; because members feel increasingly comfortable about self-disclosure, they have a better understanding about group process and the other group members, and the therapist has been asking, "How does that relate to why you are here?" and similar questions to encourage more task orientation. Nevertheless, additional focusing is essential.

It is usually possible to identify one or two central themes for each person that can become the focus of treatment interventions. Typically, the person's original goals, descriptions of outside problems, and interpersonal patterns within the group all converge to highlight the core issues. The identification of the salient themes is especially important in short-term group treatments to ensure that a majority of the group members experience the affective, cognitive, and behavioral work as productive.

Working with Affect

Trainees understand that it is necessary to plunge into affective experience, but their understanding of why this is helpful may be less clear. The most common rationale relates to catharsis, or the open expression of feelings, but as Yalom (1985) notes, "Catharsis is part of an interpersonal process; no one ever obtains enduring benefit from ventilating feelings in an empty closet" (p. 85). Furthermore, it is quite unlikely that clients will ever purge their feelings within the group again if affective expression is met with laughter and ridicule or dead silence; rather than experiencing a sense of relief, clients who face such aversive reactions are likely to feel humiliated. However, if the interpersonal consequences are constructive, clients may learn several valuable lessons: (1) that their feelings are not unique, deviant, or inappropriate, since others experience similar emotions (universality); (2) that expressing strong feelings does not lead to expected disastrous consequences (e.g., others do not hate you nor do they retaliate, and you do not lose control); (3) that feeling expression may facilitate identification, clarification, and understanding, as well as the reduction of the intensity of affective experience; (4) that there is a variety of ways, some more effective than others, for expressing strong emotional experiences; and (5) that for some clients, simply getting in touch with feelings, often defensively submerged for years, can have enormous therapeutic benefit. No doubt there are other important goals for affective expression. Overall, the benefit seems to be greater self-awareness, self-acceptance, and self-control.

While such questions as "How did that make you feel?" "What was it like to feel so depressed?" and "How does that make you feel about yourself?" may prompt affective exploration and expression, too often they foster detached description and intellectual analysis. It is much more helpful to find ways to tap into or to activate the affective experience. For example, as the person recounts painful outside situations, he or she often displays nonverbal clues to affective experience (watery or diverted eyes, changes in facial expression, quality of vocalization, etc.) A simple comment—"I have a sense that you're experiencing some of those feelings right now,"—may encourage the client to express the emotions more openly. Reflection is an often overlooked technique by beginning group therapists: "That must have caused you a great deal of pain" or "That must have felt pretty overwhelming." Often reflecting on the implications for self-esteem is productive; for example, as the person describes feeling anxious or depressed, it may be useful to comment, "That must make you feel rather inadequate," and then to explore feelings about the self more fully.

Efforts to project the person back into the situation may reactivate the feelings: "Can you picture what it was like when you were feeling so anxious?" "What would it be like if you were experiencing that feeling right now?" The what-if scenario often stimulates a reexperiencing of the painful feelings: "What if someone in the group were to treat you that way?" "How has that happened in here?" Many clinicians have underscored the importance of using here-and-now activation to evoke parallels between problems described in external relationships and those being replayed within the group. The immediacy of the affective experience, the concrete illustration of the emotional dynamics, and the capacity for other members to become invested in and to validate the emotional encounters can be a uniquely powerful experience (Ferencik, 1991; Slife & Lanyon, 1991; Yalom, 1985).

For example, over the course of many sessions a young man may have spent considerable time presenting himself as an open, caring, and sensitive partner who is having trouble understanding why he continually faces rejection in heterosexual relationships. Initially, other group members empathize with his plight, because he does seem to be getting a raw deal in many of these situations. Eventually, however, his nice-guy facade is understood as a desperate effort to win their approval, and his need to talk about his own problems, his insensitivity to the conflicts of others, and his defensiveness when challenged are increasingly experienced as unacceptable and intrusive. Soon, group members begin to reject him, as do the women in his life, because of his needy, self-centered style. He has replayed in the group the maladaptive interpersonal pattern that dominates his life outside, but now others are experiencing it firsthand and understanding the reasons for his constant rejection by others (R. Dies, in press). Confronting this repetitive, unrecognized, and self-defeating style will allow this young man to explore more constructive alternatives for fulfilling his needs.

Many beginning group therapists have not yet acquired a quick sensitivity to feeling words and thereby miss golden opportunities to encourage affective expression. The rapid flow of group events keeps them one step behind, and they are hesitant to interrupt or to return to the missed opportunity; moreover, they are reluctant to pressure clients to get into painful material. Yet many clients are extending subtle invitations or tentative feelers to see if others might be interested; indeed, they would welcome the opportunity to share their feelings (if others seem involved and willing to take similar risks). It is important to listen for affect words and to respond quickly. A client who states, "I was so hurt and confused about what happened" gives a prompt. To pick up on the confusion may lead to a cognitive focus, and to respond generically (e.g., "Can you say more about that?") may keep the focus relatively descriptive or superficial. It may be more effective to explore the hurt—"What was that hurt like?"—or the feelings behind the description—"That must have made you get pretty down on yourself."

It is also important to "think group" and to remember that there are others who have experienced similar feelings. If it is difficult for a particular member to express the emotions, it may be possible to turn to another member who can much more readily express strong emotional experiences. Once the feelings are brought to life in the room, the individual who had been struggling with the emotional expression may be able to handle more immediate affective display.

If the therapist cannot help the group members to move toward emotional exploration and expression, the level of interaction remains superficial and speculative. On the other hand, the members must also develop the capacity to step away from their feelings and to place them within a more coherent framework for self-understanding and change.

Cognitive Work

Increased self-understanding, or insight, is the goal of most forms of psychosocial intervention, but the meaning of the concept varies among clinicians. For some, insight specifically means the uncovering of unconscious conflicts stemming from childhood. For others, insight denotes any form of increased self-awareness derived from interpersonal feedback. Then there are clinicians who argue that the type of insight many clients require is not enhanced self-understanding but greater understanding of the behaviors and motivations of others. The discussion in this chapter does not require allegiance to any particular interpretation of insight.

Research clearly documents the value of self-understanding for therapeutic change (Orlinsky & Howard, 1986; Yalom, 1985), but it stands relatively mute on the nature of the insight. It is clear that any form of improved understanding has the potential to produce constructive changes in a client's capacity to cope effectively: removal of blind spots from self-perception, modification of dysfunctional and/or irrational thinking (e.g., selective inattention, catastrophizing, mind-reading, dichotomous thinking), learning specific skills, increasing understanding of others, and even acquiring general information about life. However, group treatments are especially effective in facilitating insight into the self in relationship to others.

Most people who enter therapy have done so because they wish to overcome the subjective discomfort and maladaptive interpersonal patterns that punctuate their daily lives. While significant others are often held responsible for their recurring difficulties, there is also the realization of the need for self-improvement: If they were "stronger," "more sensitive," or "more able to express feelings," they could manage their lives more adaptively. A major focus of treatment, therefore, becomes the search for the self that each client hopes to change: "Who are you?" "What is it you most want to change about who you are as a person?" "How do you keep shooting yourself in the foot in relationships?" The emphasis is on identifying the self-defeating patterns and self-fulfilling prophesies that are played out in social relationships and are often replayed in the here-and-now of group interaction. For many clients personal suffering and interpersonal ineptitude have contributed to an insidious erosion of self-esteem that can be countered and corrected in a supportive and reflective group atmosphere.

The group treatment environment becomes a hall of mirrors for self-examination. The reciprocal sharing of painful feelings and outside interpersonal conflicts and the repetition of counterproductive styles within the group provide the foundation for the interpersonal feedback or consensual validation that emerges as one of the principal sources of learning in group treatments (Yalom, 1985). Although the quality of exchange among group members is critical during the learning process, there is considerable evidence that the therapist plays a pivotal role in fostering therapeutic growth through interventions designed to promote client insight and self-understanding, that is, feedback, confrontation, and interpretation (R. Dies, 1983b, 1993, 1994). A number of general guidelines can be offered regarding the interpretive process.

1. *Interpretations that foster generalizations from interactions in the group sessions to personal experiences outside the treatment context are often regarded as most beneficial.* The demonstration of these inside–outside parallels

facilitates understanding, because the learning is immediate and concrete. The therapist frequently encourages members to search for parallels by asking, "How does that problem affect you in your interactions here?" or "Do you run into the same problems in your relationships with friends and colleagues outside?" Persistent efforts to clarify these connections provides a framework for self-examination that can be shared by other group members as they explore similar parallels in their own lives.

2. *Clients often appreciate pragmatic interpretations, advice, and instruction more than abstract analyses and "genetic" insight*, especially in short-term group treatments where the pressure of time prevents extensive exploration of earlier experiences. Flowers and Booraem (1990), for example, carefully studied four types of interpretations offered during group sessions: interpretations focused on (a) the client's impact on his or her environment, (b) patterns of behavior, (c) motives for behavior, and (d) historical causes of behavior. The interpretations that produced the greatest client change were those that addressed interpersonal impact and behavioral patterns. Others have found similar results (R. Dies, 1983b, 1994).

3. *It is useful for therapists to think about being pithy rather than profound.* Too often interpretations are framed in psychological jargon or are overly speculative, without much information to substantiate the inferences that are drawn. Interventions that are unidimensional and uncomplicated and those that are anchored by concrete examples are often more readily accepted and understood (R. Dies, 1983b). Clients need to see that what is being pointed out in their own behaviors and faulty assumptions is indeed a recurring pattern, not an inference made by others on the basis of minimal evidence.

4. *Interpretations should be offered supportively and tentatively so that clients do not feel that the therapist is judging, condescending, or playing "head-shrinking" games.* Thus, prefacing observations with qualifying comments such as "You've said several things that seem inconsistent, but maybe I'm not understanding what you mean" or "Here are a couple of different ways you might consider how that sounds to others in the group" is generally helpful. Similarly, it is often useful to simply identify contradictions between words and actions or between verbal and nonverbal expressions and then allow the client to take the first step in offering suggestions for any underlying meaning. If this step is difficult for the client, he or she might be asked if others could offer their perspectives; by granting permission for such suggestions, the client is less likely to be placed in a defensive position.

5. *Interpretations are more likely to be effective if the client is emotionally invested in the process.* Frequently, this involves the type of plunge into

affect in which the client is first encouraged to get in touch with the pain and then to reflect on the meaning of the situation. Without affective arousal, efforts to understand the personal significance of problematic thoughts, feelings, or behaviors often remain at an abstract, superficial, and/or intellectualized level of analysis.

Insight into others inevitably occurs during group treatment, as clients openly discuss feelings, thoughts, motivations, and actions. For most group members, this opportunity for intensive sharing and self-exploration with contemporaries is unique, and for many it is their first experience of interpersonal closeness and intimacy.

Working on Behavioral Change

For many clinicians, fostering insight and catharsis has much greater appeal than any direct efforts to promote behavioral change, since it is assumed that modifications in behavior naturally occur with increased understanding and emotional relief. Other therapists, however, believe that it is often "easier to act yourself into a new way of thinking than to think yourself into a new way of acting" (R. Dies, in press), and they direct considerable effort toward interventions that encourage behavioral practice, both within and between treatment sessions. These efforts are thought to provide increased opportunities for learning, which, in turn, furnish a foundation of increased self-awareness.

Participation in the complex social "microcosm" (Yalom, 1985) of group psychotherapy inherently demands the learning of social skills that many clients lacked before they entered treatment: interpersonal compromise and confrontation, active listening, commitment and responsibility, honest communication and expression of feelings, and so forth. Indeed, the acquisition of these social skills is often reported as a major accomplishment during treatment (Yalom, 1985), and there is evidence to suggest that clients who learn these behaviors most effectively are also the ones who derive the most benefit from treatment (Tschuschke & Dies, 1994).

Much of the research on group treatments involves short-term interventions designed to teach specific problem-solving skills. Indeed, dozens of treatment manuals have been written in recent years that provide concrete guidelines for how therapists can model or demonstrate effective interpersonal behaviors and then reinforce group members in their efforts to modify their own actions accordingly (R. Dies, 1994). While a majority of these programs are based on cognitive-behavioral models of treatment, the clinician does not have to be a behaviorist or a psychodramatist to make effective use of action-oriented techniques. A few examples of the available options may be helpful.

One alternative is simply to suggest that the client practice a new behavior within the group. Thus, with encouragement and in the context of a supportive group climate, an unassertive client might be asked to express her feelings more spontaneously or in a more forceful manner, to "see how it feels," with the understanding that such experimentation in the group provides an excellent opportunity for feedback from others. Acquiring a new skill (e.g., becoming more assertive) is a little like learning how to walk; you may fall a few times, but if you pick yourself up and try again, it gets easier each time. A client who has made an insensitive comment can be asked to think of alternative ways of expressing himself that might be less offensive to other group members and then supported in his efforts to do so. Another client might be given several alternatives and requested to select one for practice. In each case, it is useful to explore the assumptions that clients have made about their behavioral choices: "If I assert myself, they might not like me"; "If I don't come on strong, they'll think I'm weak"; "If I show my feelings, I'll make myself too vulnerable."

The faulty assumptions that govern many maladaptive behavioral strategies can then be explored openly and their self-defeating nature challenged directly. For many clients, a basic message is that the "what if" is worse than the "what is," that is, that anticipated negative outcomes are far worse than the actual consequences. Many clients also discover that choices to avoid short-term disadvantages often generate even more significant long-range problems. For example, our unassertive group member can be shown that although she circumvents potential criticism from others by not talking, the ongoing self-abuse for being so passive is much more costly in terms of lowered self-esteem and chronic unhappiness. Clients can be helped to understand the "neurotic paradox," that by shying away from fearful circumstances, they are also avoiding the very situations that might help them to unlearn their counterproductive patterns. Similarly, clients might learn that their efforts are backfiring. The person who remains quiet to avoid being rejected by peers is, by her silence, generating the very interpersonal outcome that she is attempting to prevent. Clients often discover that the most effective way to change maladaptive behaviors is just to bite the bullet and to change them. Group treatment provides a safe forum in which to experiment with new behaviors.

Clients could be invited to demonstrate rather than talk about a problem that occurs outside: "Can you show us how you did that?" "What did you actually say? Can you repeat the words here and now in the same way?" A simulation of the outside circumstance might reveal that rather than coming across as sensitive and caring, as the client hoped, other clients react to the critical and judgmental part of the message. In this fashion, the discrepancy between intentions and interpersonal impact can be explored. In other instances, a formal role play can be enacted (Kipper, 1991) and the client encouraged to practice different ways of relating. For example, "Why don't you try that right now? I'll be your boss and you come in and ask me for the raise. How would you do that?" The use of role plays allows members to practice new behaviors and to receive guidance from peers for further understanding and refinement. The group setting affords an arena of safety for trial-and-error learning to occur. The use of members as resources substantially enhances this learning process, as clients are more likely to learn from their fellow participants because of their perceived commonalities rather than from leaders who are viewed as more distant models (R. Dies, 1993).

It is also useful to provide homework assignments for interpersonal projects that can be attempted between treatment sessions (Ellis, 1991). It has been argued that one of the major reasons for the success of cognitive-behavioral approaches to short-term group therapy is the assignment of specific between-treatment tasks (Graff, Whitehead, & LeCompte, 1986). Therapists of other theoretical orientations have also found that clients who work most between sessions to build on the interpersonal experiences acquired within the group are the ones who derive the most benefit from treatment (Lieberman, Yalom, & Miles, 1973). In generating assignments to be applied in their clients' natural environments, it is important for therapists to think in terms of "successive approximation" toward a desired goal (K. Dies & R. Dies, 1993). In other words, start with assignments that are less threatening and gradually increase the level of expectation. This arrangement may facilitate a benign cycle, in which earlier accomplishments improve confidence to face more difficult assignments. As members report on their efforts to implement new behaviors in their everyday lives, successes are reinforced, failures are accepted for the effort they represent, and members are helped to understand how to improve their performance. Practice in the real world has the potential to generate supportive responses from significant others, which is much more reinforcing than the feedback from the therapist or fellow group members. Moreover, transfer of learning of new skills is enhanced.

Most clients readily accept homework assignments if they understand the rationale for their introduction, recognize that other group members are interested in the activities and have their own opportunities for such practice, and know that the assignments are pertinent to their problems. Once beginning group psychotherapists discover the powerful effects such social engineering efforts can have on their clients' well-being, they too feel much more accepting of these intervention strategies.

Cotherapist Communication and Group Focus

It is rather artificial to divide the affective, cognitive, and behavioral work of group therapy into separate sections in this chapter. During the working phase of treatment the therapist intervenes at multiple levels, with different clients benefitting as a function of their own personality styles. Some need to "try it out," whereas others have to "see how it feels" or to "think about it." Most gain increased self-understanding from each type of intervention, both directly and indirectly (through observational learning).

By this stage of group treatment, cotherapists have become much more effective working together as a team. They have learned how to read each other's signals, and they feel more comfortable openly discussing goals for interventions during the sessions. Collaboration rather than parallel play or competition is much more common. Nonetheless, many cotherapists are reluctant to communicate more personally with each other during the sessions. Despite the popularity of the notion that cotherapists serve as effective role models for group members, there is little evidence to support this claim (McNary & Dies, 1993). The modeling that does occur appears to be more in terms of the working alliance or professional collaboration, not of personalized interactions involving self-disclosure or the expression of here-and-now feelings. Yet the willingness to confront and work through personal differences regarding leadership, to share feelings of support and admiration, and to express a range of normal reactions to relationship issues can be effectively integrated into the working phase of group development (R. Dies, 1977, 1983b; R. Dies, Mallet, & Johnson, 1979; McNary & Dies, 1993): "Beth [cotherapist], I feel envious at times because you're so supportive of others. I wish I was able to be so open." Openness between coleaders can foster similar exchanges among group members and enhance the potential for more constructive interpersonal feedback.

The format for individual work among clients varies in different groups. Although a turn-taking style is adopted by members of some treatment groups, a pattern in which several members are working on a common core issue, such as depression, self-esteem, or victimization, is more usual. There may be a "lead client," but others will participate actively in the process. The working through of personal and interpersonal problems unfolds over time, with recurring cycles of intensive work on central problems. The work on individual issues typically follows a "plunge–reflect" cycle (Yalom, 1985) over the course of many sessions, as clients explore different facets of their problems and as outside events stimulate even further material for therapeutic exploration.

Understanding and change are generally gradual and their amount and nature depend on the time frame of the treatment contract. Long-term groups allow for exploring the deeper significance of current problems and broadening the members' understanding of their presenting symptoms and maladaptive interpersonal styles. Time-extended treatments also furnish other opportunities not available in brief forms of treatment: The strength of the interpersonal bond among members may be more substantial, and the inevitable termination of individual clients may precipitate a focus on loss and the need to integrate newcomers. However, the framework of this chapter is short-term group treatments, and in this context, termination generally means the conclusion of the group experience for all of the participants.

TERMINATION

The amount of time devoted to a discussion of termination depends on how long the group has been convening; for short-term group treatments several sessions should be set aside for this type of work. Generally, the therapist(s) must once again assume the responsibility for structuring the sessions to ensure that each client has the opportunity to address final issues. It is also necessary to adopt a more group-centered perspective to highlight the shared group-level reactions that clients invariably experience as the group draws to a close. At least four tasks are important during the final phase of group development (K. Dies & R. Dies, 1993).

First, it is necessary to wind up unfinished business. On a personal level, this may entail the recognition of learning yet to be completed, which in turn may require a review of each person's original goals (R. Dies, 1983a; R. Dies & K. Dies, 1993b). On the group level, the process may involve the closure of unresolved interpersonal issues, for example, tensions over a previous disagreement or unverbalized feelings of appreciation for support received during a recent discussion of an outside crisis. Members who feel that an agenda item is incomplete may, in light of the group's imminent conclusion, feel pressed to address the issue and seek personal and interpersonal relief. The leaders' invitation to share unfinished business legitimizes its expression.

The second integral aspect of the ending stage of group psychotherapy is helping members plan what they are going to do after treatment is over. For some clients, the short-term group experience has provided sufficient learning and self-understanding to consider their treatment completed. For these group members, the therapist encourages a discussion of how to generalize the coping skills learned during the sessions to daily transactions in the real world. "What if your spouse begins to treat you that way again?" "What will you do if you begin to doubt your abilities again?" These types of questions prompt clients to remain focused on problem-solving skills and to anticipate how to handle difficulties before they arise. Group members are helped to understand that periodic setbacks are likely and that the best way to calibrate improvement is in relationship to their level before treatment and over blocks of time (e.g., month to month).

For clients seeking to continue treatment, multiple alternatives exist that require little elaboration at this point. Ironically, many trainees are reluctant to tell clients, "I think you need more therapy," even though they believe it, because they are afraid to hurt their clients' feelings or embarrass them in front of their peers, especially when other clients have "graduated" successfully. Yet most clients who have participated in 10 to 20 sessions of treatment are well aware of their progress and of the work that remains to be accomplished; thus, those who need more therapy usually volunteer for it rather than waiting for the therapist to recommend it. Therapists should be aware of available alternatives and be prepared to help clients follow through with future arrangements.

Once clients have made and shared their tentative post-treatment plans, they are in a better position to face the emotional implications of ending their present group experience. At this point, it is the leaders' responsibility to encourage group members to work through termination. Clients' reactions to termination will vary according to their degree of investment in the treatment process, but the therapists' role is to help members cope with feelings of loss regardless of their nature or intensity. Leaders must be cautious not to allow members to bog down in excessive emotionality or to remain withdrawn and closed off from their affective experiences. Nor is this a time to attempt extensive individual therapeutic work or to open new issues. The presentation of new material must be identified as work for future treatment, so that the therapist can more effectively guide the members into processing their current emotional experiences.

A group that has been supportive and within which significant connections have been made among the members may wish to deny the fact that the group will soon end. Someone may propose that the members continue to meet at one of their homes or at least to hold a reunion or party at some future date. A task-oriented member might even begin collecting telephone numbers to ensure that the meeting takes place. Other group members may intellectualize or gloss over their emotional reactions to the group's ending and engage in excessive cognitive processing of events in an effort to flee them. In the face of diversionary tactics, therapists must maintain a clear focus on the inevitability of the termination. Some members may indeed see each other in the future, but the group as it now exists will cease to be and the experiences that members shared cannot be recaptured.

The meaning of this loss must be explored. What has the group experience meant for each person? What are the feelings about coping without this support system? How is this loss like others that have been experienced? Can clients express what they really feel? The final sessions thus become an opportunity for additional learning about honest and direct communication with others. During this period of intense emotions, it is necessary for therapists to be aware of their own issues around experiences of loss. Some therapists hide behind their professional role, reluctant to share their own sense of loss. They too do not know how to say goodbye. It is especially difficult for leaders and clients who have had different feelings toward each participant. They may feel comfortable about saying to some, "I have really felt close to you and will miss what we have been able to share," less comfortable saying to others, "I regret that we weren't able to make a better connection, but I have felt good about your efforts to share." Differential feelings toward others is a fact of life, and learning how to express these reactions openly and sensitively is a valuable lesson to be learned, for therapists as well as clients.

Learning how to cope with loss at the group's ending is vital to successful treatment. Mastering this period is a product of helping members to consolidate their cognitive and emotional work. Cognitive processing focuses on generalizing skills learned in treatment to other people, places, and life situations. Emotional processing involves interpersonal aspects of what the group has meant to each member. Therapists help members to integrate their cognitions and feelings, emphasizing the interpersonal experiences that have fostered learning. During this period, the therapist seeks to orchestrate continued interaction among members, avoiding individual reports of change and emphasizing interpersonal aspects, to underscore the behavioral changes that represent the outcome of client self-disclosure and feedback throughout the group's life cycle. The significance of interpersonal relationships is what sets group treatment apart from other forms of psychotherapy.

The closing interventions by the therapist often provide rituals through which clients may express their feelings. Whether through a moment of silence, a certificate of participation, or group or individual hugs, leaders help members to bring closure to their group experience. One particularly poignant symbolic ritual of ending, for example, involves a ball of yarn that is passed from member to member, each person holding onto a piece of yarn that passed through his or her hand (K. Dies &

R. Dies, 1993). As the ball is exchanged by clients, there develops an intricate pattern of yarn that represents the varied interactions among the members. In the closing step of this exercise, the members snip the yarn that binds them together, severing the connection and marking the termination of the group. The members take with them the pieces of yarn that remain in their hands, symbolizing the learning they have acquired during the treatment process.

CONCLUSION

Hundreds of books and thousands of articles offer recommendations for conducting group treatments effectively. The suggestions are influenced by each author's theoretical predilections, professional experiences, and personal style. Although my list of basic leadership principles no doubt reflects an equal assortment of idiosyncratic features, it is my hope that the guidelines outlined in this chapter have sufficient generalizability to be useful for practitioners representing many different views.

The field of group psychotherapy has matured considerably since its inception over eight decades ago (R. Dies, in press), but we still have much to learn about the unique potential of this treatment modality. Just as there are many ways to learn through participation in group treatments, there are also various ways to intervene successfully. While it is unlikely that a generic model of group treatment can be adapted to fit all treatment settings equally well, the principles provided in this chapter have been found to be serviceable in a wide range of clinical contexts.

REFERENCES

Bahrey, F., McCallum, M., & Piper, W. E. (1991). Emergent themes and roles in short-term loss groups. *International Journal of Group Psychotherapy, 41,* 329–345.

Bernard, H. S., Drob, S. L., & Lifshutz, H. (1987). Compatibility between cotherapists: An empirical report. *Psychotherapy, 24,* 96–103.

Beutler, L. E., Crago, M., Arizmendi, T. G. (1986). Research on therapist variables in psychotherapy. In S. L. Garfield & A. E. Bergin (Eds.), *Handbook of psychotherapy and behavior change* (3rd ed., pp. 257–310). New York: Wiley.

Dies, K. R., & Dies, R. R. (1993). Directive facilitation: A model for short-term group treatments, Part 2. *The Independent Practitioner, 13,* 177–184.

Dies, R. R. (1974). Attitudes toward the training of group psychotherapists: Some interprofessional and experience-associated differences. *Small Group Behavior, 5,* 65–79.

Dies, R. R. (1977). Group therapist transparency: A critique of theory and research. *International Journal of Group Psychotherapy, 27,* 177–200.

Dies, R. R. (1980). Group psychotherapy: Training and supervision. In A. K. Hess (Ed.), *Psychotherapy supervision: Theory, research and practice* (pp. 337–366). New York: Wiley.

Dies, R. R. (1983a). Bridging the gap between research and practice in group psychotherapy. In R. R. Dies & K. R. MacKenzie (Eds.), *Advances in group psychotherapy: Integrating research and practice* (pp. 1–26). New York: International Universities Press.

Dies, R. R. (1983b). Clinical implications of research on leadership in short-term group psychotherapy. In R. R. Dies & K. R. MacKenzie (Eds.), *Advances in group psychotherapy: Integrating research and practice* (pp. 27–78). New York: International Universities Press.

Dies, R. R. (1985). Leadership in short-term group therapy: Manipulation or facilitation? *International Journal of Group Psychotherapy, 35,* 435–455.

Dies, R. R. (1991). Clinician and researcher: Mutual growth through dialogue. In S. Tuttman (Ed.), *Expanding domains of psychodynamic group therapy* (pp. 379–408). Madison, CT: International Universities Press.

Dies, R. R. (1992a). The future of group therapy. *Psychotherapy, 29,* 58–64.

Dies, R. R. (1992b). Models of group psychotherapy: Sifting through confusion. *International Journal of Group Psychotherapy, 42,* 1–17.

Dies, R. R. (1993). Research on group psychotherapy: Overview and clinical applications. In A. Alonso & H. I. Swiller (Eds.), *Group therapy in clinical practice* (pp. 473–518). Washington, DC: American Psychiatric Press.

Dies, R. R. (1994). Therapist variables in group psychotherapy research. In A. Fuhriman & G. Burlingame (Eds.), *Handbook of group psychotherapy* (pp. 114–154). New York: Wiley.

Dies, R. R. (in press). Group psychotherapies. In A. S. Gurman & S. B. Messer (Eds.), *Major systems of psychotherapy.* New York: Guilford Press.

Dies, R. R., & Dies, K. R. (1993a). Directive facilitation: A model for short-term group treatments, Part 1. *The Independent Practitioner, 13,* 103–109.

Dies, R. R., & Dies, K. R. (1993b). The role of evaluation in clinical practice: Overview and group treatment illustration. *International Journal of Group Psychotherapy, 43,* 77–105.

Dies, R. R., Mallet, J., & Johnson, F. (1979). Openness in the coleader relationship: Its effects on process and outcome. *Small Group Behavior, 10,* 523–546.

Dies, R. R., & Teleska, P. A. (1985). Negative outcome in group psychotherapy. In D. T. Mays & C. M. Franks (Eds.), *Negative outcome in psychotherapy and what to do about it* (pp. 118–141). New York: Springer.

Egan, G. (1986). *The skilled helper* (3rd ed.). Monterey, CA: Brooks/Cole.

Ellis, A. (1992). Group rational-emotive and cognitive-behavioral therapy. *International Journal of Group Psychotherapy, 42,* 63–80.

Ferencik, B. M. (1991). A typology of the here-and-now: Issues in group therapy. *International Journal of Group Psychotherapy, 41,* 169–183.

Flowers, J. V., & Booraem, C. D. (1990). The frequency and effect on outcome of different types of interpretation in psychodynamic and cognitive-behavioral group psychotherapy. *International Journal of Group Psychotherapy, 40,* 203–214.

Graff, R. W., Whitehead, G. I., & LeCompte, M. (1986). Group treatment with divorced women using cognitive-behavioral and supportive–insight methods. *Journal of Counseling Psychology, 33,* 276–281.

Kipper, D. A. (1992). Psychodrama: Group psychotherapy through role playing. *International Journal of Group Psychotherapy, 42,* 495–521.

Kivlighan, D. M. (1985). Feedback in group psychotherapy: Review and implications. *Small Group Behavior, 16,* 373–385.

Kivlighan, D. M., Corazzini, J. G., & McGovern, T. V. (1985). Pregroup training. *Small Group Behavior, 16,* 500–514.

Kivlighan, D. M., & Quigley, S. T. (1991). Dimensions used by experienced and novice group therapists to conceptualize group process. *Journal of Counseling Psychology, 38,* 415–423.

Koss, M. P., & Butcher, J. N. (1986). Research on brief psychotherapy. In S. L. Garfield & A. E. Bergin (Eds.), *Handbook of psychotherapy and behavior change* (3rd ed., pp. 627–670). New York: Wiley.

Lieberman, M. A. (1983). Comparative analyses of change mechanisms in groups. In R. R. Dies & K. R. MacKenzie (Eds.), *Advances in group psychotherapy: Integrating research and practice* (pp. 191–213). New York: International Universities Press.

Lieberman, M. A. (1989). Group properties and outcome: A study of group norms in self-help groups for widows and widowers. *International Journal of Group Psychotherapy, 39,* 191–208.

Lieberman, M. A., Yalom, I. D., & Miles, M. B. (1973). *Encounter groups: First facts.* New York: Basic Books.

Livesley, W. J., & MacKenzie, K. R. (1983). Social roles in psychotherapy groups. In R. R. Dies & K. R. MacKenzie (Eds.), *Advances in group psychotherapy: Integrating research and practice* (pp. 117–135). New York: International Universities Press.

MacKenzie, K. R. (1987). Therapeutic factors in group psychotherapy: A contemporary view. *Group, 11,* 26–34.

MacKenzie, K. R. (1990). *Introduction to time-limited group psychotherapy.* Washington, DC: American Psychiatric Press.

Mayerson, N. H. (1984). Preparing clients for group therapy: A critical review and theoretical formulation. *Clinical Psychology Review, 4,* 191–213.

McNary, S. W., & Dies, R. R. (1993). Cotherapist modeling in group psychotherapy: Fact or fantasy? *Group, 17,* 131–142.

Melnick, J., & Woods, M. (1976). Analysis of group composition research and theory for psychotherapeutic and growth-oriented groups. *Journal of Applied Behavioral Science, 12,* 493–512.

Orlinsky, D. E., & Howard, K. I. (1986). Process and outcome in psychotherapy. In S. L. Garfield & A. E. Bergin (Eds.), *Handbook of psychotherapy and behavior change* (3rd ed., pp. 311–381). New York: Wiley.

Roback, H. B., & Smith, M. (1987). Patient attrition in dynamically oriented treatment groups. *American Journal of Psychiatry, 144,* 426–431.

Roller, B., & Nelson, V. (1991). *The art of co-therapy: How therapists work together.* New York: Guilford Press.

Slife, B. D., & Lanyon, J. (1991). Accounting for the power of the here-and-now: A theoretical revolution. *International Journal of Group Psychotherapy, 41,* 145–167.

Tschuschke, V., & Dies, R. R. (1994). Intensive analysis of therapeutic factors and outcome in long-term inpatient groups. *International Journal of Group Psychotherapy, 44,* 185–208.

Vinogradov, S., & Yalom, I. D. (1989). *A concise guide to group psychotherapy.* Washington, DC: American Psychiatric Press.

Yalom, I. D. (1985). *The theory and practice of group psychotherapy* (3rd ed.). New York: Basic Books.

• FOUR •

PRINCIPLES OF GROUP THERAPEUTIC TECHNIQUE

Kenneth Porter

Teaching psychotherapeutic technique is a paradoxical endeavor, for technique is a secondary issue in the practice of psychotherapy. When the therapist is working best, technique is unconscious. Therapists are not divided into separate portions within themselves—mind and heart, technique and feeling. As the British group analyst Wilfred Bion put it, they are "beyond memory, understanding and desire." They function as integrated wholes.

Yet viewed from without, as therapists express themselves to their patients, technical regularities can be observed. To some extent, these regularities can be taught and learned until ultimately they disappear into the seamless web of the therapist's integrated conscious and unconscious functioning.

This chapter considers six of the most important aspects of group psychotherapeutic techniques: general principles, resistance, transference, countertransference, primitive group dynamics, and the negative effects of group therapy. Each section except the first is followed by exercises of imagination. Readers may wish to write down their preferred course of action before reading the suggested solutions in order to increase the value of the exercises.

GENERAL PRINCIPLES OF GROUP LEADERSHIP

The main task of the patient in group therapy is to learn how to be in relationship. Since relationships lie at the heart of human existence, most difficulties that bring patients into treatment can be ameliorated through the medium of the group.

The main task of being in a relationship is to learn to appropriately balance the needs of oneself with the needs of the relationship. To emphasize only the needs of the individual in a relationship produces two or more individuals engaged in parallel play. To emphasize only the needs of the relationship produces codependency. To appropriately balance the two produces a relationship.

This being said, one can proceed to address the main task of the group therapist, which is to help group members learn how to relate. This means that the group therapist and the members of the group must learn to balance the needs of each individual with the needs of the group.

Using this format for understanding, it is possible to divide the technical tasks of the group therapist into two large categories: those that involve the healing of individual members and those that involve the development and maintenance of the group.

Attending to Individual Needs

Facilitate the Expression of Feelings in Words

This is the basic curative mechanism of all psychotherapy, whether group or individual. It is based on the principle that humans are verbal animals, that a major way we can be ourselves is through talking. The act of verbalizing a feeling is a way of knowing that feeling, releasing it from purgatory. As we talk we overcome splits within ourselves. Since for most patients the major splits within themselves have involved the disowning of feelings, the process of expressing feelings in words helps patients repossess these feelings and this makes patients whole again. It is important for the therapist to convey that all feelings, no matter how crazy, primitive, or socially inappropriate, are acceptable to express in words in the group.

Focus as Much as Possible on the Here-and-Now

Effective psychotherapy requires a balanced consideration of a patient's past life, current life dilemmas, and here-and-now interactions in therapy. Since our society erects major taboos against individuals revealing the true content of their minds in social situations, the major resistance in therapeutic situations tends to be toward discussing the here-and-now. Hence, the therapist's main efforts need to be toward facilitating this level of expression.

Interpret Unconscious Experience

Experienced therapy group members develop great facility in interpreting deep aspects of each others' lives, but when all is said and done this remains the task of the group psychotherapist. Though less important than in individual therapy, the empathic communication to patients of the therapist's understanding of aspects of their experience that are outside of their awareness is a mainstay of group therapeutic technique, especially in group therapy that has a psychoanalytic orientation.

Attending to Group Needs

Maintain the Therapeutic Frame of the Group

The group therapist must forge the group into an effective therapeutic instrument. This requires the same careful attention to the therapeutic frame as in individual therapy. Although after a while group members take over responsibility for much of their therapy, the maintenance of proper group structure remains the responsibility of the therapist. Attendance, punctuality, fees, new members, termination, confidentiality, and acting out all require careful and ongoing consideration.

Make the Group into the Main Therapeutic Agent

Whenever possible the therapist should encourage the group or an individual member to do therapeutic work. This can be accomplished by directing comments to the group such as "What is going on in the group now?" "What does John need at this point?" "Why is the group not dealing with this issue?"

Stimulate and Guide Group Interaction

This noninterpretive intervention is crucial to the maintenance of effective therapeutic group process. The leader can question individuals, agree, nod, give verbal support, and in many verbal and nonverbal ways encourage the flow of interpersonal interaction. Generally speaking, the more psychologically impaired the members of the group are, the more the leader needs to engage in this type of behavior. But in even the most sophisticated group, the stimulation of group interaction remains the task of the leader.

Educate the Group

Many group leaders underemphasize the crucial importance of explicitly educating group members in the process of doing group therapy. No patient enters treatment, whether individual or group, automatically understanding how to behave in order to derive the maximum benefit from the process. It is the task of the group leader to educate group members in the norms of effective therapeutic group behavior in the following three ways:

- *Educate group members to relate to each other in mutually helpful ways.* What distinguishes group therapy from individual therapy, of course, is that the treatment is taking place in a social context: the presence of other patients. This means that to the basic dictum of "putting feelings into words" must be added "in a mutually helpful way." In this way the art of relationship is explored in the group context.
- *Establish the norm of exploring problems rather than blaming.*
- *Establish the distinction between the constructive expression of anger and the acting out of anger through verbal sadism (abuse).*

RESISTANCE

Resistance is the central issue in psychotherapy. Whether it is explicitly recognized or not, all therapy must deal with resistance as the fundamental obstacle—and pathway—to change.

What is resistance and why does it exist? Human beings automatically move away from emotional pain as they do from physical pain. Operating according to this pleasure principle, from the earliest moments of life we seem to separate ourselves from, dissociate, repress, or split off experience that is painful. This protects us, but it also leads to internal fragmentation rather than internal wholeness.

Severe alienation from aspects of internal experience can be healed by psychotherapy. But as the therapist attempts to bring into awareness previously dissociated painful material, the patient identifies the therapist and therapy itself with the unacceptable experience. A defense against internal experience is transformed into resistance to the interpersonal process of psychotherapy. Hence, the therapist's ability to deal effectively with resistance can make the difference between successful and unsuccessful treatment.

Although it is time-honored, the term "resistance" is in many ways unfortunate. It implies a model of therapy that is incorrect. The term suggests that the main impetus in therapy comes from the therapist and that the patient is resisting it. The term in everyday language also connotes a conscious and intentional process, whereas much of resistance is unconscious. Finally, the term usually implies something negative. On the contrary, however:

- *Resistance is a normal reaction to growth*. Growth requires the integration of previously dissociated experience, which is painful and naturally resisted.
- *Resistance is needed for self-protection and healing*. Human beings naturally alternate between periods of openness and periods of self-protection. Self-protection is necessary to shield the organism from being overwhelmed with rawness, experience, change, and anxiety. Resistance, if it does not rigidify, is therefore as healing as openness.

Nature of Group Resistance

Resistance can be a group-wide phenomenon as well as an individual phenomenon. It is a fascinating and crucial aspect of group as opposed to individual functioning that certain phenomena that are outside the awareness of each individual can operate on a group basis. This occurs because the individuals in a group experience a psychological entity that is larger than themselves—the group—as having reality and are able to unconsciously project into that entity aspects of their own experience that they find unacceptable. An example of this is group resistance, of which all the individuals in the group are unaware.

Certain signals indicate when a group resistance is occurring:

- *Clinical intuition*. The group therapist has a sense that the group is "stuck." A reliable indication is feelings in the therapist of boredom or irritation with the whole group.
- *Pervasiveness*. In the usual mode of group functioning, on any issue there will be a diversity of thoughts and feelings. But when the group is in resistance, the entire group seems to act in a uniform way that feels unnatural—for example, everyone is angry, everyone is silent.

- *The group persistently tolerates an individual member's resistance.* This indicates unconscious participation in the individual's resistance by the group.
- *Timing.* Group resistance often occurs at times of crisis in the group—when members enter or leave, when the therapist or key members are absent, or when new material is introduced.
- *Group behaviors.* Certain behaviors of the group suggest resistance: passivity on the part of the group (waiting for the therapist to do something); constant fighting; one-to-one relating in the group, either among members or between a member and the therapist, that excludes the rest of the group; superficiality of relating (chit-chat, intellectualization); silence that persists; acting out on a groupwide level (lateness, absences, missed payments, extra-group socialization in defiance of the therapist's recommendation); over-focusing on one member, either through scapegoating or monopolization.

Treatment of Resistance in Group Therapy

Give priority to resistance. Since resistance is a normal part of the human psyche and of the growth process, it should not be viewed as an obstacle to be overcome in order to get to the "real" therapy. Often the feelings in the resistance itself are the heart of the therapy.

Accept resistance. Do not attack resistance. Resistance occurs because patients feel that parts of themselves are unacceptable. But since patients also identify with these disowned parts, when patients resist they will also feel that *they themselves* are unacceptable.

For this reason, when the therapist treats a patient's resistance as unacceptable the patient feels even more unacceptable and hence becomes even more resistant. The solution is for the therapist to accept the resistance and explore it with the patient, this enables the patient to begin to accept what is internally taboo.

Maintain an awareness that resistance can be unconscious. The resistance that is blatantly obvious to the therapist may be totally outside the awareness of the patient.

Maintain resistance at optimal levels. The more resistance is dissolved by the therapeutic process, the more anxious a patient becomes. But the optimal level of anxiety is not the same as the maximal level, since too much anxiety paralyzes a patient. On the other hand, too little anxiety causes the therapy to stagnate. So when resistance is high in a group, the therapist should vigorously pursue it.

Deal with resistance before exploring any underlying feelings. When patients are in a state of struggle with the therapist, they are less open to the therapist's deeper interventions. First confront patients; ask them to step back and observe that they are blocking something out. Then clarify how the blocking is occurring (e.g., arguing or withdrawal). Then explore the deeper feelings (what is being blocked).

Educate the group members to the concept of resistance and to the goal of helping each other dissolve their own resistances.

Deal with resistance in order of clinical importance:

1. Resistances related to violence or suicide
2. Resistances that threaten the continuity of the group
3. Resistances that threaten the continuity of an individual's treatment
4. Sudden group resistance
5. Sudden individual resistance
6. Ongoing group resistance
7. Ongoing individual resistance (character traits)

Exercises

1. A new patient in group therapy sits silently for a number of sessions, although she is clearly troubled. The group therapist silently speculates on the meaning of her silence and on the proper intervention. In the meantime the group makes occasional mild attempts to engage the patient. She says only a few words, and then the group members move on to other issues. The group therapist should

    a. ask the patient if she wishes to talk.
    b. ask the group why they are allowing the patient's silence to continue.
    c. allow this to continue, as it demonstrates the characterological pattern of the patient.

Discussion. This example illustrates a number of the complexities of dealing with resistance in group therapy. Finding an appropriate intervention in the situation is not simple. Ordinarily response b is the best procedure. It accomplishes two things at once: It both reaches the patient's resistance and also teaches the group about their responsibility for the therapeutic process. But suppose this patient is insecure about the therapist's concern. Then it might be more useful to temporarily forego the advantage of response b and use response a to solidify the working alliance with the patient. If the silent patient is firmly ensconced in the group, response c might be most appropriate. If the patient is not yet integrated into the group, allowing her to sit silent too long might lead to overwhelming feelings of isolation and rejection and to the patient dropping out of treatment.

2. A patient well along in group therapy persists in coming late for apparently iron-clad reasons. In other respects, this member is clearly committed to the group. From knowledge of the patient, the therapist knows that tardiness is a pattern in other areas of the patient's life that he has had difficulty confronting. In the group the patient plays a role of elder statesman. The group has great respect for him and never addresses any possible deeper aspects of the patient's tardiness. The therapist should

- a. ask the group why they have not addressed the issue with the patient.
- b. not intervene, as this is the group's responsibility.
- c. interpret the lateness to the patient as probably related to underlying feelings, and encourage him to explore that probability.

Discussion. Option b runs afoul of both an individual and a group resistance that seem to be underway. Option c could of course be followed, but it leaves out what might be most interesting of all—why the group is tolerating the lateness and what it is about the patient that might be inducing them to do so.

TRANSFERENCE

Resolving transference is crucial to all forms of psychotherapy. To the extent that therapy is psychoanalytically oriented, resolving transference is the core of the therapeutic process. But even when therapy is not primarily psychoanalytic in nature, the manner in which transference is managed has a profound effect on the success of the treatment.

Why is transference so crucial? First, for most individuals, the key that determines how much satisfaction they experience in their lives is the quality of their relationships. Since relationship stands in such a central place in our lives, it is also the most powerful lever in therapy for opening an individual's dysfunctional system.

Second, what is most powerful in relieving pathology is what is most emotionally real to the patient. In the therapy office the most emotionally present relationships for patients are usually those with the therapist and fellow group members. The greatest power to change behavior will derive from working with these relationships in the here-and-now, including their distortions through transference.

Why does transference occur? Transference is the experience of another person as someone from our past. As human beings we seem unable, without great effort, to fully live in the present. Fully living in the present would mean to live each moment with maximum appropriate intensity, to then let it go, and to then proceed to the next moment. But we seem unable to perform this letting go. Instead, we carry over feelings—desires and fears—to the next moment. This basic mechanism of transference prevents us from cleanly living the next moment without distortion.

Transference thus prevents full interpersonal intimacy. To the extent that transference is present we are not able to fully relate to other people as the people they truly are.

Types and Characteristics of Transference

There are two basic types of transference in therapy:

- *Traditional concept of transference.* We experience the other person as a whole person, separate from us, but confused with someone from the past.
- *Transferences intended to repair self-esteem.* In this type of transference the other person is experienced not as a separate person but as someone whose accepting presence we need to make a part of ourselves, in order to repair an insecure sense of self-esteem.

Transference in group therapy has several characteristics:

- *Multiple levels.* Transference may be to fellow group members, to the therapist, or (very crucial and often overlooked) to the group as a whole.
- *Multiple targets.* In group therapy multiple transferences by a patient are possible at the same time—for example, mother, father, siblings, grandparent.
- *Familial aspects.* A patient may have a transference to the whole group as a family in either the positive sense ("This group is like the family I never had!") or the negative sense ("You're just like my family!").
- *Dilution.* Because of the presence of multiple targets for transference, any one particular transference, for example the transference to the therapist, may be diluted and therefore may be easier to resolve.

- *Ease of resolution.* Difficult transferences are often easier to resolve in group therapy than in individual therapy for many reasons: patients see others' different transferences; patients have the support of other patients to express frightening feelings; patients can make use of other members' insights.

Working with Transference

In working with transference in the group setting, the therapist must consider the following factors: the nature of the treatment (ego-supportive or uncovering); the nature of the transference (traditional or self-reparative); the timing of the intervention; the means or route of the intervention (should the intervention be made directly to the patient or to the group?); and the importance of working through.

Nature of the treatment. Therapy that is ego-supportive tends to strengthen the ego through education, reduction of shame and guilt, and the replacement of primitive with higher-level defenses. It does not emphasize making unconscious material conscious. Uncovering (or insight-oriented) therapy tends to reduce ego defenses in order that unconscious experience may be integrated into the ego. In the course of therapy most patients need both approaches at different times, but at any given moment one approach tends to predominate.

Group therapists should vary their intervention according to the nature of the work they are doing with any given patient. Supportive treatment, generally appropriate for more impaired patients, tends to interpret negative transference quickly, before it becomes a major obstacle in treatment. For example, if a patient is perceiving the therapist or a group member inaccurately, the therapist might point this out immediately. Positive transference is usually left uninterpreted to form a basis for the patient's therapeutic progress.

Uncovering treatment, on the other hand, is usually used with healthier patients. In this approach, both negative and positive transference are usually allowed to develop. The full power of the treatment generally lies in deeply working with both aspects of transference when they are fully developed.

Nature of the transference. In accordance with current thinking on psychoanalytic technique, transferences in which the primary need is for the therapist's acceptance are best dealt with by not interpreting their unconscious meaning. The therapist or group should rather try to provide, insofar as realistically possible, the heretofore missing acceptance and, when this is not possible, should empathically clarify the realistic limits of the situation. Traditional transference, on the other hand, is best dealt with by helping the patient understand its deeper meaning.

Timing of the intervention. Much of the technique of working with transference lies in the art of timing. All transferences need to be allowed to develop to some extent, which requires that the therapist communicate an attitude of acceptance toward the transference. Obstacles (resistances) to the expression of transference, such as embarrassment, shame, and guilt, need to be explored and accepted.

Mistakes in timing tend to be of two types. Intervention that is too early produces an overintellectual experience at best; at worst it may embarrass the patient and drive the transference underground. On the other hand, interpreting transference too late may permit the establishment of a strong dysfunctional pattern that is hard to dislodge.

As in the dyadic setting, the therapist acts most productively when transference intensity and anxiety are optimal: not too high and not too low. Usually the best time to intervene is after a good working alliance has been established and when the transference is strong enough to begin to interfere with therapy (i.e., it is becoming a resistance) but has not yet become extremely intense.

Who should make the intervention? Generally speaking, in this area as in other areas of group treatment, it is best for the group to do as much of their own as possible. The therapist may encourage all group members to express their transferences, may contrast the different transferences, may stimulate group members to support each other in expressing frightening or painful transference feelings, and may ask the group to interpret a particular member's transference. When necessary there is nothing wrong with the therapist making the interpretation, but working through the group should at least be attempted.

Working through. Transference is clarified and ultimately resolved through a process of repetitive exploration. In group therapy a crucial component of the working through process—missing from the therapist's armamentarium in individual treatment—is the opportunity for the patient to practice ways of behaving that are alternatives to older transferential patterns. The group becomes a laboratory in which the patient experiments with healthier ways of relating, including effective self-assertion, constructive expression of anger, effective expression of dependency needs, and less guilt-ridden and anxiety-ridden expression of sexual feelings.

Exercises

1. A female group member is in love with her male group therapist and discusses it in the group. As the situation develops, the transferential aspects of the patient's feelings are clear to the therapist and even alluded to by the patient, but the strength of her feelings does not diminish and

in fact intensifies. The group seems slightly thrown by the situation and basically allows the patient to discuss her feelings with the therapist in the group without much intervention. The therapist should

   a. allow the situation to develop, in order to more fully explore the transference.
   b. say nothing about the situation, so as not to embarrass or humiliate the patient.
   c. encourage the group to respond to the situation.
   d. encourage the patient to express these feelings in the group.
   e. offer the patient individual therapy.

Discussion. This thorny and challenging situation offers a number of opportunities and pitfalls for the group therapist. Options a and b, though seemingly considerate and theoretically sound, run a great risk of allowing a transference pattern to become entrenched, which will not be helpful to the treatment. Option e might or might not be helpful, but it might well exacerbate the situation and might represent a resistance or countertransference problem on the part of the therapist; it certainly should not substitute for dealing with the issue in the group. Option c is by far the safest and best course.

2. A group member at an advanced point in therapy is obviously very committed to her treatment. Her pattern is to present a problem in group and become intensely emotional, taking 30 to 45 minutes to fully express many emotions with great honesty and depth. As she thus regresses to an earlier level of development, she seems to experience the group as a nurturing mother. The group admires her and tries to give her the support she seeks. On the outside her life has improved somewhat but she remains stuck in certain crucial areas. The therapist should

   a. support this pattern, as it represents a reparative transference to the group as a whole that can heal a crucial narcissistic wound.
   b. directly interfere with the patient's taking so much group time by interpreting her transference directly to her.
   c. ask the group what this pattern means, whether it is useful for the patient, and whether they should support it.

Discussion. This was an actual case of mine, and I first tried option a. After a while it became apparent that although it may have been constructive at first, the behavior was unfair to the rest of the group and also seemed to be a resistance on the part of the patient. I next tried option b, partly to signal to the group that they did not need to tolerate unproductive behavior but partly also out of frustration. The situation only truly started to resolve itself productively when I tried option c several times.

PRIMITIVE GROUP DYNAMICS

Groups affect the deepest areas of the human psyche and give rise to certain primitive psychological processes that form the warp and the woof of group therapeutic process. These reactions in themselves are neither harmful nor helpful. When properly understood and directed by the group therapist, they can be a source of great healing power. But when misunderstood or misused, they can lead to significant negative clinical effects on patients, groups, and therapists themselves.

Primitive Group Processes

Regression. Members of any group tend to experience a mental entity called "the group" and to give it reality, merging their individual egos with it in the way infants merge their egos with their mothers. This leads to a state of ego regression, in which the egos of the individual group members and the entity of the group are not distinguishable on an unconscious level and the individual is operating on a developmental level that dates from an early stage of life. This state of regression can be extremely useful clinically, since it enables the group process to reach down and heal the deepest aspects of character distortion. But regression can facilitate other processes, such as projective identification and scapegoating, that can be dangerous if not handled correctly by the therapist.

Projective identification. The unconscious regressive state that occurs in groups facilitates a unique process known as projective identification. In this process an individual internally disowns a feeling and then projects the disowned feeling onto another individual, while retaining a sense of connection with the disowned feeling. The recipient of the projective identification experiences the disowned feelings that are being received but may not be clear whether these are his or her own feelings or those of the individual who is engaged in the projection.

Projective identification forms the basis of much of the group process in a group therapeutic setting. Group members are continuously experiencing and expressing feeling states that arise not only from their own internal psychological processes but also from the emotions that are being induced in them by other group members engaging in projective identification.

Scapegoating. Projective identification has a variant that is crucial for the process of group therapy—scapegoating. In this form of projective identification, the members of a group engage in two unconscious processes. First, they project an unacceptable feeling into a group member, a feeling whose existence is denied within themselves. Usually a group member is chosen whose character difficulties match the projected feeling and who is therefore a willing recipient for the projection.

Second, the group members project hostility into the entity of "the group" while disowning it in themselves. The group then acts out an attack on the scapegoat. However, the individual group members do not experience themselves as engaged in an attack; "the group" seems to be the responsible agent.

Management of Primitive Group Processes

Regression. Like anxiety and resistance, regression needs to be maintained by the group therapist at an optimal level that is neither maximal nor minimal. Too little regression produces flat, superficial treatment; too much regression leads to acting out and treatment disruption.

Generally speaking, therapists can control the level of regression in a therapy group by varying their own interventions. When a group is experiencing too little regression, the therapist can try either silence or deeper interpretations to increase the regressive process. Correspondingly, when regression is too great, more conscious verbal activity, in the form of explanations, reassurance, support, and guidance, tends to decrease the regressive pull of the group process.

Projective identification. On a minute-to-minute basis, projective identification forms the matrix of much of group therapeutic interaction. Early in the life of a therapy group, it is therefore useful for the therapist to explain the mechanism of projective identification to the group so that they can use the concept as a tool for understanding each other's internal lives.

Awareness of projective identification is also useful during moments of individual or group resistance. Particularly at times when an individual or the entire group seems stuck in what to the therapist appears to be an off-target reaction, the therapist should consider the possibility of exploring projective identification needs with the group.

Scapegoating. The process of scapegoating can be particularly pernicious to the success of a therapy group. Whenever one member is strongly and persistently criticized by the other members of the group, the leader should check for the possibility of scapegoating. When present, scapegoating needs to be quickly interrupted and interpreted.

But how does the therapist distinguish scapegoating from the crucially important therapeutic process in which the group usefully challenges the dysfunctional behavior of a group member? First, in a useful therapeutic interaction the confrontation has the tone of caring, even when anger is present. In scapegoating, by contrast, a hostile quality can be discerned. Second, when the confrontation is therapeutic the patients who are the focus of the challenge usually change positively over time and indicate that they feel helped. In scapegoating there is a "stuck" quality to the group interaction. Finally, in useful confrontation group members may be able, when it is helpful, to acknowledge the presence within themselves of the difficulty they are pointing out in the member on whom they are focusing. In scapegoating the group members are in denial about some significant aspect of themselves.

The group therapist also needs to bear in mind that scapegoating frequently represents a defense against anger toward the therapist. This occurs when leaders communicate that they are unavailable for confrontation and group members therefore displace their unacknowledged negative feelings toward the easier target of a fellow group member.

Exercises

1. A patient who tends to intellectualize reports in a flat tone of voice an incident at work in which he was clearly mistreated and whose significance he seems not to appreciate. In fact, this is one of many such instances that the patient has discussed in the group, without perceiving an apparent pattern. Instead of being directly helpful to the patient, the group members become quite angry at him, which makes him defensive, and the group begins to attack him. The group therapist should

   a. protect the patient by pointing out to the group that they are being critical.
   b. inquire into the group's critical stance, with the possibility in mind that the group may, through projective identification, be picking up and amplifying the patient's own unconscious anger.
   c. join with the group in the opportunity to work on a dysfunctional aspect of the patient's character.

Discussion. In this situation it is always tempting for the group therapist to go to option c, but it is usually more useful to begin with option b. This often leads to option c but in a more natural and less jarring manner.

2. In his first session, a new patient in a very experienced therapy group presents a very arrogant stance. He acts as if he has no problems, says he is only coming to the group because the therapist suggested it,

and maintains that the group members are obviously far more disturbed than he is. The group therapist is aware that the patient is a highly insecure man with deep feelings of inferiority who compensates by a grandiose posture. The group becomes infuriated and incisively begins to attack the new patient's character. The group therapist should

    a. consider the possibility of scapegoating.
    b. support the process, hoping that it will help the new patient learn about the ways in which he interacts with others.

Discussion. In this quite common situation, option b usually leads to a group dropout. The task here is not individual therapy but integrating the new patient into the group. Most experienced groups should be able to discern that the patient's behavior is a defense against anxieties about being a new group member. If the group does not attend to this, the likelihood is that they are feeling angry at the leader for introducing a new member and displacing it onto a scapegoat. This is often the more fruitful line to pursue.

COUNTERTRANSFERENCE

The term "countertransference" has been used in two ways in the field of psychotherapy—to refer to the reactions of the therapist to a patient's transference and, more broadly, to refer to all the reactions of the therapist to the totality of a patient's communications. The second sense seems more useful.

Types of Countertransference

Countertransference in the broadest sense falls into two categories. *Objective countertransference* refers to the therapist's reactions to a patient's communications that would be roughly similar in all therapists engaged with the patient. *Subjective countertransference*, on the other hand, refers to the reactions that occur within the therapist due to his own idiosyncratic emotional and personality patterns.

    Countertransference reactions can be either symmetrical or complementary. *Symmetrical reactions* are those that are identical to the feelings patients are denying. For example, patients who are denying their anger may induce angry feelings in the therapist. In contrast to this, *complimentary reactions* are those that are reactive to the feelings that patients deny. An example of this would be patients denying anger and inducing either fear or guilt in the therapist.

Objective countertransference is of crucial importance in group therapy. It is based on the phenomenon of projective identification, with the leader being the target of the projective identification process. This leads to the therapist's developing feelings within himself that correspond to the feelings being denied by one or several group members. These feelings can be a rich source of data for the therapist about the internal functioning of the members of the group.

Prevention and Management of Countertransference Errors

Countertransference mistakes in group therapy may he based on either subjective or objective countertransference reactions, and they are similar to those that occur in individual treatment. In addition, certain other countertransference mistakes are unique to group therapy, including the reactions of the group therapist to the group as a whole. At times a therapist is intimidated by a group and becomes passive, overpermissive, or unable to provide leadership or overcome a resistance. At other times therapists become authoritarian and overcontrolling toward a group, at times out of fear that they may be overwhelmed. These reactions may occur because the group unconsciously represents a feared individual or family situation in the past of the therapist.

Aside from the usual recommendations for adequate supervision and peer consultation, the most reliable guidelines for preventing and resolving countertransference mistakes include the following.

Pay particular attention to whether a countertransference error is present. When treatment with a particular patient is in difficulty, a reliable though at times painful procedure is for the group therapist to overtly request input from the group regarding the difficulty. If the leader is genuinely receptive and the group has been democratically led, most groups will be unsparingly but appropriately honest about their leaders' shortcomings.

Acknowledge mistakes without reservation. Once an error has been recognized, if it has been severe or prolonged, an apology may be called for. Then the therapist should return to the more traditional work of therapy, which in this case is to elicit the patient's further feelings, including the patient's anger, and to help the patient resolve any resistances to the full expression of these feelings. It is not the easiest of tasks for therapists to work on eliciting anger toward themselves in spite of a patient's natural inclination to protect them.

Two pitfalls present themselves. One is for the therapist, out of a natural sense of guilt and defensiveness, to settle for a superficial expression of feeling by the patient, to not fully explore the patient's pain hoping that the issue will disappear. Every opportunity must be taken to raise the issue repeatedly with the patient when it is present in latent form in the clinical material. In the case of severe countertransference mistakes, weeks, months, or even years of investigation may be required before a full resolution can occur. The other pitfall is for the therapist to become overapologetic or the target of excessive hostility or verbal abuse by the patient, which only exploits the patient once again, this time in the service of the therapist's excessive need for punishment.

Therapists may fear that too frank an admission of error or too deep an exploration of the patient's anger will lead the patient to terminate treatment or even (where the mistake has been severe) initiate legal action. The opposite is the case. Major difficulties arise primarily when the patient senses a significant error that the therapist does not acknowledge. Perhaps surprisingly, patients are quite forgiving, even of major countertransference problems, if they sense genuine pain in the therapist and if they are encouraged to fully explore their own pain without encumbrance by defensiveness or masochism on the part of the therapist.

Countertransference errors are not to be regarded as simply unfortunate occurrences. To the extent that patients view their therapists as parents, it can be a rare and salubrious experience to have a parent who is honestly willing to admit to faults. The countertransference error, when fully explored, allows for a depth of feeling on the part of the patient that carries the therapy far beyond the point of being just an intellectual exercise. When the error is fully acknowledged the possibility exists for an experience that may be rare in the patient's life in or out of treatment.

Exercises

1. A woman who has been in therapy for a considerable period of time complains that her therapy has not helped her at all, that she is in fact worse since she started treatment, and that her therapist does not care for her. The therapist is aware that this patient had a cold, competitive mother and a depressed and withdrawn father. The therapist interprets the patient's material transferentially, but the complaints only intensify and the patient states that she wishes to stop treatment. The therapist should

    a. more vigorously interpret the patient's transference, and attempt to use material from other group members to support this position.

    b. ask the patient what she specifically feels the therapist has done wrong and why.

    c. accept the patient's proposal that she stop treatment since the therapy seems to be at a standstill.

    d. ask the group members what they think is going on.

Discussion. In this actual situation the therapist first tried option a unsuccessfully, then silently considered option c. Under these circumstances, option d will be useful only if the therapist conveys to the group a genuine interest in the group members' true opinions, regardless of whether they are flattering to the therapist. In this case a combination of options d and b led to major movement. It became apparent in succeeding group sessions that a major problem had existed in the relationship between patient and therapist of which the therapist had been unaware. The patient then made very significant improvements.

2. A group of mostly schizoid men has great difficulty working at a deep therapeutic level. The group therapist often feels bored and critical of the superficial nature of the work and spends long periods of time saying nothing. After the one remaining woman in the group terminates, the group therapist repeatedly tries to add new female members one or two at a time, but on three different occasions the new members leave the group within 6 months. On one occasion the therapist starts the group 30 minutes late. The group therapist should

  a. add a large number of new female patients at once.
  b. explore with the group the possibility of resistance to having women in the group.
  c. attempt to add to the group individuals of either sex with differing personality styles.
  d. terminate the group.
  e. continue to run the group as an all men's group.
  f. explore with the group why he started the group late.

Discussion. In this case options a, b, and c, all quite reasonable, did not produce the desired effect. In desperation the therapist considered option d. When, for lack of an alternative, option e evolved, the therapist became aware that he had been participating in a group resistance and had in fact become as withdrawn and prone to overintellectualization as the group members. He also realized that he had been expecting the group members to function at a higher level than was possible. When the therapist forgot the group's starting time, the situation came to a head. Option f led to a frank discussion in which the group members told him that as the group therapist he was too withdrawn and uninvolved. Recognizing the truth of this the therapist changed his approach, and from that point on the group started to jell as an all-male group, becoming more lively and interesting to the therapist as well as to the members.

NEGATIVE EFFECTS OF GROUP THERAPY

The negative effects of group therapy have not received the attention they deserve. This is because group therapists, like all human beings, tend to turn away from considering their mistakes. But just as the medical doctor uses the postmortem examination to identify and correct his limitations, so too can group therapists explore, prevent and treat the negative outcomes that result from the practice of their craft.

General Causes of Negative Effects

Aside from countertransference errors, the usual sources of negative effects in group therapy lie in certain common technical mistakes:

- *Insufficient attention to boundary issues*: punctuality and attendance of patients, punctuality and attendance of the therapist, fees, new members, terminations.
- *Insufficient activity on the part of the group therapist in educating the group* to appropriate norms of therapeutic group behavior and adoption of a supposedly "analytic" attitude of passivity. This is especially harmful when the therapist fails to distinguish between the constructive verbal expression of anger, which should be encouraged, and the acting out of sadism through verbal abuse, which needs to be quickly prevented.
- *Insufficient cultivation of the group as a therapeutic instrument*, insufficient stimulation of group interaction, and overreliance on one-to-one therapist–patient interaction in the group.
- *Insufficient attention to group resistances and improper management of the primitive group dynamics* of regression, projective identification, and scapegoating.

Causes of Specific Negative Effects

Specific negative effects in group therapy include:

- *Premature dropouts from group therapy*, which usually arise from the following sources:

  1. A patient is selected who is inappropriate for group therapy (examples are the patient who is too paranoid, narcissistic, or borderline or the patient for whom the referral to group therapy represents an unclear attempt to resolve a resistance in the individual treatment).

2. A patient is added to a group that is inappropriate for that patient.
3. The group therapist makes a technical mistake in the early stages of a patient's participation in the group, for example, allowing the new patient to be scapegoated.

- *Groups that fail to develop* usually reflect one of the following difficulties.

  1. A group resistance is present that has not been identified and resolved by the leader.
  2. Faulty group composition has occurred, such as insufficient diversity of personality styles.
  3. Faulty selection has allowed a patient with destructive psychopathology, such as sociopathy, to enter the group.

- *Emotional harm to patients in ongoing treatment* may occur as a result either of shortcomings in the therapist's knowledge or skill or of countertransference difficulties.
- *Emotional harm to the group therapist* is a rarely discussed but important occurrence. Common causes are:

  1. The failure of a group under a beginning group therapist who does not receive sufficient supervision, which undermines the therapist's feeling of competence.
  2. A sense of excessive guilt when significant emotional harm occurs to a patient, if the therapist takes the event as a reflection of his or her total competence.
  3. Not recognizing that an individual, subgroup or entire group is engaged in hostile acting out toward the leader, leaving the leader with feelings of being devalued.

Danger of Abuse in Group Therapy

In rare instances a negative effect of group therapy may reach such proportions as to merit the term "abuse." Such is the case when (1) a patient is persistently harshly criticized or scapegoated by the group or by the therapist, (2) the therapist exploits a patient practically or financially, or (3) major boundary violations occur, such as sexual contact between therapist and patient.

Abuse can arise in the group setting when two circumstances come together. The first is a therapist with major unconscious countertransference or characterological difficulties and an intense need to control or hurt others, who in addition is an appealing, brilliant, or otherwise charismatic individual. The second is a patient with profound unsatisfied narcissistic or dependency needs that make him or her both vulnerable to exploitation and unable to recognize accurately situations where mistreatment is occurring.

When they come to light, such situations need to be openly discussed in professional settings, thus educating potential patients, current patients, and therapists to a greater level of awareness, paving the way for therapists to expose their work to the scrutiny of their peers in preventive efforts, and stimulating the development of the professional mechanisms that are needed to reveal and resolve such instances of inappropriate professional behavior.

Exercises

1. A very experienced patient who has always been unusually responsible and dedicated to therapy and his group suddenly walks out of a session and subsequently announces to his therapist that he is terminating therapy on the spot, without explanation. He turns and leaves the office in spite of the therapist's urging him to stay and discuss the situation. One year later he requests an individual session. With considerable feeling he reveals that during his entire treatment he felt seriously hurt and misunderstood in major ways. The therapist should

   a. explore the validity of the patient's complaint and the possibility of continuing treatment based on a new understanding of the previous work.
   b. interpret the patient's leaving as acting out and explore why he could not directly tell the therapist how angry he was.
   c. interpret the patient's transference.

   Discussion. Under circumstances such as this, option a is the only viable possibility. It is at times possible even under such extremely negative circumstances for the treatment to continue and even to reach hitherto unsuspected depths of healing.

2. A patient who is himself a therapist undergoes group therapy and finds himself in a situation where the group therapist, though seemingly brilliant and helpful, has actually behaved in an abusive manner. The treatment ends, but as the patient develops perspective on the situation, he realizes that in his own clinical work as a therapist he has inadvertently identified with his former therapist and as a result has introduced significant distortions into the treatment of a number of his own patients. The therapist should

   a. bring the situation up with the relevant patients, explain what has occurred, and reveal his own history so his patients will understand the total situation better.

   b. look for indications in his patients' clinical material that they have felt hurt or angry at his past behavior and carefully explore these instances, remaining open to the possibility of acknowledging error once the patients have had the opportunity to fully explore and express their feelings.

   c. say nothing to his patients but work within himself to become aware of how he has erred so that he can refrain from similar behavior in the future.

Discussion. The two major pitfalls here are the two extremes—saying nothing to patients, which is probably inadequate for dealing with a difficult situation, or confessing everything, which interferes with meeting the patient's needs. Option b is usually the best course and can produce, under the circumstances, surprisingly therapeutic results.

CONCLUSION

This chapter has discussed certain key technical issues in the conduct of group psychotherapy. We have reviewed general principles of technique and explored the subjects of resistance, transference, countertransference, primitive group dynamics, and the prevention of negative results in group therapy.

Generally speaking, attention to technique is only one aspect of the development of the group therapist. In the course of their careers, most group therapists devote a significant portion of their professional time to their own emotional maturation, including experiences as patients in group therapy, and to exploration of the theory (as opposed to the technique) of group therapy. Nonetheless, especially in the early stages of their training and at times of difficulty in their careers, group therapists can enhance their conscious capacity to heal the patients who come to them for professional help by considering the guidelines of therapeutic technique.

• FIVE •
DIFFICULT PATIENTS AND CHALLENGING SITUATIONS

Harold S. Bernard

This chapter focuses on the responses therapists can make to particular patients and situations that often emerge in the context of ongoing group treatment. Before beginning to discuss the specific issues that constitute the bulk of this chapter, it is important to acknowledge some factors that might affect the approach a therapist takes toward "problem" situations.

One such factor is the nature of the patient population with which the therapist is working. Specifically, how high-functioning is the group as a whole? The answer to this question has important implications for the nature of the working contract. Higher-functioning patients are capable of doing a different kind of psychological work than are lower-functioning patients. Specifically, higher-functioning patients are suitable for insight-oriented groups which work toward individual change, including the modification of characterologic patterns. By way of contrast, support groups aim at helping individual members to adapt to and cope with their life circumstances as effectively as possible.

Another factor is the phase of a group's development (Chapters 2 and 3). Thus, if a difficult situation emerges early in a group's history, the therapist decides what tack to take on the basis of its probable impact on the group's effort to establish a sense of cohesion. If the same dilemma emerges at a later point in the group's life, the therapist takes a different tack according to the developmental issue occupying the group at that time.

For purposes of conceptualizing the dimensions of therapeutic contract and phase of group development, it is helpful to think in terms of the following:

	Supportive	Insight-oriented
Early		
Transition/differentiation		
Working		
Termination		

Let me indicate how this grid can be useful. In all groups, obstructions periodically emerge that hinder the group's work to a greater or lesser extent. A therapist would consider the variables represented in this grid, among others, in deciding what tack to take. In a support group at any stage in its development, the therapist might opt to remove the obstruction as quickly as possible, either because the group is not capable of doing so itself or because the group's accomplishment of this task would not facilitate the achievement of the goals of the group. Similarly, the therapist might opt to attempt to resolve the problem in an insight-oriented group if the group is in such an early stage of development that the therapist is not confident the group can manage the situation successfully. However, if the group is farther along, the therapist might take a less proactive stance and allow the situation to fester for a period of time, either because the group is clearly capable of managing it or because the therapist believes the group *might* be capable of handling it and that it would be desirable for individual members or the group as a whole if it succeeded in doing so. Such working through of problems can be among the most powerful experiences in insight-oriented group work.

The nature of the working contract and the stage of a group's development determine the way the roles of therapist and patient are defined. Specifically, how much is the therapist the "leader" of the group? What are the responsibilities of the group patient? To what degree are the patients responsible for themselves and for each other (and the therapist)? These matters are *not* obvious, and must be addressed during the pregroup phase (see Chapters 1 and 2).

One or more of the factors I have just touched on can affect the approach a therapist would take in a difficult situation. Because the underlying beliefs and theoretical perspective a therapist carries into the treatment situation profoundly influence how the therapist responds to almost anything that emerges in the group, it is important for me to briefly articulate my approach to group treatment. I am an interpersonally oriented group therapist in the tradition of Yalom and others (Yalom, 1985). While my understanding of patients is primarily informed by psychodynamic thinking broadly defined, I tend to be an active and goal-directed therapist who makes every effort to tackle a group's dilemmas so that its basic work (namely the giving and receiving of interpersonal feedback) can begin or resume as quickly as possible.

With this framework, let us begin to look at the struggles group therapists often confront.

DIFFICULT PATIENTS

The first section of this chapter will focus on a variety of difficult patients that frequently test group therapists. While not exhaustive, the range of patients described will give the reader a sense of the variety of challenges that groups, and group therapists, must confront.

The Silent (Withdrawn) Patient

When a patient is withdrawn in a group, the dilemma for the therapist is to determine when and how the issue should be addressed. How much time should such individuals be given to "find their voice," that is, to begin participating actively in group discussion? Is it simply a matter of the patient not being sufficiently comfortable to participate, or should another explanation be considered: for instance, that it is an attention-getting device? If the issue is to be addressed, should the therapist simply do so himself or herself, or should the therapist somehow attempt to facilitate the group's doing so?

The following describes a prototypical scenario with a silent patient:

Isabel, a 43-year-old single woman, presented for group therapy quite ambivalently from the outset: Her individual therapist thought it would be a good idea and she decided (after many months) that she was willing to try it, though she was not at all sure it was what she wanted or needed. Though she was quite interpersonally isolated, she contended that she had made her peace with being alone and that in many ways she preferred it to being involved with others, which had always resulted in pain and disappointment for her in the past.

Unsurprisingly, Isabel said very little during her first two weeks in the group. When asked why she was in group, she spoke vaguely about her therapist thinking it would be a good idea, and no one pushed her very hard for more specificity. The few comments she volunteered were exclusively thoughts and observations about others, with no personal content whatsoever.

The therapist's decision was to address the issue early (by Isabel's third session) and to do so in different ways at different times thereafter. Working with a patient such as this requires persistence and flexibility of approach; it is usually not a matter of exploring the silence once and thereby resolving the problem.

The therapist primarily used three approaches.

1. He asked Isabel to talk about her experience of being in the group and her thoughts about revealing things about herself. It is important to note that the therapist did not directly request that she talk about herself before she was ready to do so; he never wavered from the notion that the decision about whether to talk about herself was hers and hers alone to make. However, he did broach the issue so that it became a public issue within the group rather than one Isabel was dealing with only internally.

2. He periodically asked others what thoughts and feelings they found themselves having about Isabel. This approach can be useful as long as the therapist is not implicitly asking group members to "kick" the patient in question. What can be mobilizing is the patient hearing the variety of feelings generated in others at different stages as her silence/withdrawal continues.

3. He talked about his own feelings as he continued to struggle with how to work most effectively with Isabel. There are certainly limits to therapist self-disclosure. For instance, if a therapist feels rage, despair and hopelessness in relation to a particular patient, it is probably best to suppress such feelings as long as one continues to hope to find a way to work effectively with someone (and perhaps even when one has given up). However, to describe one's struggle to find a way to engage such a patient is to talk out loud about something everyone in the group knows is occurring. Such interventions serve as models for how all members of the group might grapple with their relationships with each other and with the therapist and how they might help silent patients learn about the reactions they elicit in others.

Of course, none of these strategies guarantees success with this kind of difficult patient. They do suggest, however, that therapists have a variety of tools to attempt to get treatment with these patients untracked.

The Monopolizing Patient

The patient who dominates group discussion presents an equally difficult challenge to the group therapist. Monopolization is often thought of as cropping up in the early stages of the life of a group; the reason is that the tendency to monopolize is associated with a particular personality (or character) style, and since character is consistent, the tendency to monopolize usually emerges early. However, such a tendency usually persists and remains a problem at every stage in a group's development.

Whereas silent patients are mostly a danger to themselves in terms of their ability to remain in a group and benefit from it, a monopolizer is a threat to the group as a whole. If the process of monopolization continues over a number of sessions, as it often does, it can quickly lead to patients becoming hopeless about the group, resigned, and disengaged. They come to think of the group as simply a place where Mr. or Ms. X holds forth, not a place where a session will be useful to them. This is why it is so important to tackle the problem sooner rather than later.

Following is a description of a therapy group in which a monopolizer took over and threatened the group's continued viability.

> Rich is a 48-year-old single male who is openly homosexual. He has been unattached all his life; his sexual relations have always involved mutual masturbation with strangers in public restrooms. He is extremely bright and highly obsessive, with great dexterity in language; in fact, he speaks five languages fluently.
>
> Rich dominated discussion from the beginning of the group. When he talked about himself he did so in great detail; at first others were charmed by him and impressed by his extraordinary articulateness. When he commented on what others said, he often began by seeming to be responsive to them but invariably got so involved in what he was saying that in effect the focus switched to him. While it was clear that others tuned out soon after he began speaking, the group was stymied as to how to deal with Rich for a number of weeks.

This kind of situation presents the therapist with a frequently encountered dilemma: How much does the therapist take the lead in dealing with a particular problem as opposed to letting the group find its way to a solution? Let me suggest strategies for both of these approaches.

One reason a therapist might deem it necessary to take the lead in a situation like the one described is that group members often experience patients like Rich as formidable and are too timid to confront them. It is incumbent on the therapist not to be intimidated by any patient. If the therapist decides to take the lead, he or she might say something like "I'm aware that Rich has been talking much more than anyone else here, and yet it seems difficult for anyone to acknowledge this and to talk about their feelings about it." While the therapist is not expressing first-person feelings about Rich's monopolization, he or she is speaking to the issue and indicating that it can be and should be addressed. In this way, the therapist is indicating that he or she is not intimidated and encouraging others to feel similarly.

If this approach does not work, an even more direct statement by the therapist might be required. While discussion by a therapist of what he or she feels about a particular patient can be dangerous, it can be very powerful and, when used at propitious moments, necessary to move a group forward. In this instance, a therapist has the option of saying something like "Rich, my frustration has been building as you've taken up so much of the group's time in the last few weeks. I've found it hard to know how to address this and thus have not said anything up until now, so I know I have some responsibility for letting it happen. I wonder how aware you are of the extent to which you have been the center of attention and what it has been like for you."

Such an intervention focuses the group on the process of what has been occurring in its interaction. One of the possibilities is that the floodgates of frustration will be opened, putting Rich in danger of being scapegoated. It is imperative that scapegoating be avoided, and strategies for avoiding it will be addressed in the "Scapegoating" section of this chapter. Even short of this, however, is the danger of the loss of the therapeutic alliance with Rich. The threat of this possibility is why it is so risky to intervene in this way, especially early in a group's life when the alliance may not be firmly established, and it is especially risky with monopolizers, who are often narcissistic personalities, whether diagnosable according to the criteria of the *Diagnostic and Statistical Manual of Mental Disorders*, third edition, revised (DSM-III-R; American Psychiatric Association, 1987) or not, and thus often oblivious to the role they have assumed in the group and its impact on others.

In order to avoid these dangers, the therapist should attempt to do two things. First, it is important to portray what is going on in the group as a process that everyone, including the therapist, has some responsibility for, rather than as something the monopolizer is doing to the group. Second, the therapist must convey interest in understanding the monopolizer's experience: what the monopolizer is trying to accomplish, what needs underlie the behavior, and so on. In other words, the therapist, while acknowledging frustration, must view what is occurring in the group the way he or she construes everything else: as an opportunity for all members to learn. Conveying this attitude minimizes the likelihood that the patient will feel punished and uncared about.

If the therapist, instead of taking the lead, wishes to encourage the group to do the work required, he or she can ask the group to consider what is occurring in the here-and-now; that is, to switch its focus from whatever content is being discussed to the process that is unfolding. If group members are able to address their thoughts and feelings about what is occurring, the therapist's job is to facilitate discussion and to make sure the group focuses on its process as long as necessary.

The decision about how proactive the therapist needs to be in intruding into the process of monopolization should be based on an assessment of the degree of danger the group is in: The greater and more immediate the danger, the more proactive the therapist needs to be. Often therapists first attempt to get group members to take the lead, and then, if this does not work, intervene themselves.

The Boring Patient

While this problem sometimes overlaps with monopolization, it is in fact distinctive. Sometimes patients monopolize without being boring (Rich, the patient described in the previous section, was experienced by most as fascinating to listen to), and sometimes patients are boring without monopolizing.

Following is an example of a boring patient.

Doug, a 36-year-old single, male bond broker, was experiencing significant professional reverses at the time he was being treated in group. His activity level in the group was about the same as the other group members. What was distinctive about his participation was the style and content of his contributions. He was stuck in every realm of his life and was experienced as never saying anything new: He was making less and less money, he was not happy in his putative "relationship" with a woman he saw periodically but was not inclined to do anything about it, and he was enraged with his mother and his brother and seemingly unable to make any headway on these fronts either. His style of presentation was deadly: He spoke in a monotonous drone that had no life to it and that turned others off as soon as he began speaking.

From the point of view of the therapist the first step is to realize that the patient's boringness is what needs to be addressed and, in fact, is more important to explore than whatever content he might be discussing. Unlike the monopolization problem, the issue is not particularly urgent and does not need to be addressed immediately; however, it must be addressed at some point if Doug is to benefit from the group experience. It is the kind of issue that can be avoided indefinitely because it is difficult to talk about: Group members shy away because they feel that to discuss it can be very invalidating and potentially hurtful. But as with many such issues, addressing it often turns out to be less catastrophic than feared: Doug, for example, knew that he was experienced as boring. In fact, in the example, when the group finally was able to talk about the issue, Doug volunteered that his nickname at his place of work was "Dead Man."

Once again, the therapist has options for helping a group begin to discuss such subject matter. It is best when the group is able to undertake such work on its own: It is a sign that the group has progressed to the point where it understands the therapeutic task and can take responsibility for doing the hard work that makes group therapy so powerful. Of course, therapists are not an unimportant presence when this occurs; on the contrary, they must be particularly alert to how the recipient of the feedback is responding. If the patient is taking it well (i.e., seems to be hearing it and considering it), the therapist may need to say little or nothing. On the other hand, if the patient seems to be overwhelmed by the feedback, the therapist must be ready to intervene in an empathic way without negating or otherwise undercutting what has been said. One way to do this is to say something like "My sense is that Doug is no longer able to hear what people are saying and to make constructive use of it. Doug, while I think that much of what has been said to you is worth your consideration, perhaps we have gone about as far as we can with this today. What do you think?" The effort is to communicate empathy without negating the potential value of the feedback that has been offered.

When group members are not able to find a way to address the issue on their own, the therapist can always take the lead by making note of others' nonverbal reactions when the boring patient begins to speak. Invariably, group members fidget, look away, or exchange glances of exasperation or bemusement. Asking group members to put their feelings into words is usually all that is required to get them into the issue. If this does not work, the therapist may need to firmly break the ice by saying something like "It seems hard for people to talk about the monotone Doug uses when he talks about himself." Once again, the therapist needs to be alert to the potential for scapegoating and to the possibility that the patient will feel injured in a way that threatens the therapeutic alliance and must be prepared to address these dangers if necessary. Nevertheless, these risks must be taken at times or the potential payoffs from a group therapy experience will not be realized.

The Therapist Helper

Patients can help the group therapist in a variety of ways. They can take the lead in initiating discussions that seem therapeutically useful. They can initiate feedback to other patients that moves the therapeutic process forward. They can even praise the therapist for all his or her good works. However, such contributions may be at the expense of dealing with the issues that brought the individual into treatment.

Sometimes therapist helpers are difficult to spot, especially when the therapist wants or needs assistance. They seem to be involved in the group and working hard, and they are apparently pleased with what they are getting from the experience.

The following illustrates the dilemmas in dealing with therapist helpers in groups.

Sidney, a 28-year-old male, presented for treatment with concerns about his relationship with his father, for whom he had worked since graduating from college. He felt unrecognized and unappreciated by his father and uncertain about what, if anything, he could or should do about it.

At the beginning, Sidney became the de facto leader of the group. Sometimes he brought in rich material to work on, and at other times he took the lead in being responsive to others. While many of his comments could simply have been construed as contributions to the ongoing work of the group, they also unmistakably revealed a concerted effort to please the therapist. Every initiative the therapist took was supported in one way or another by Sidney, and other members soon began to see Sidney as paired with him. Sidney quickly developed a strong commitment to the group and talked about how important each and every member, the therapist, and the group as an entity had become to him. Finally, he praised the therapist regularly for being brilliant, talented, and humane, and he became very defensive of the therapist when one or more members challenged him in some way.

Dealing with patients like Sidney clearly presents some countertransference challenges. Specifically, it is easy to be seduced by such individuals, both because they are contributing so much to the group and because it is appealing to be appreciated and respected. When praise is crassly obsequious, it is much easier to deal with than when the patient focuses specifically on the attributes one feels most proud of and when the patient's style is matter-of-fact rather than obviously crafted to win the therapist's favor.

Once again the challenge for the therapist is twofold: he or she must first recognize the pattern, then develop a strategy for addressing it. The therapist must get past the gratitude and come to see that the patient is living out a pattern in relation to authority figures in his life that must be critically examined if therapeutic movement is to occur. Sometimes other patients can see the pattern more clearly than the therapist; it is

important for the therapist to be humble enough to acknowledge missing things, sometimes for long periods of time.

Once the pattern becomes clear, the therapist should look for a
propitious time to address it. However, as with the other patients and
situations described in this chapter, there is more than one approach.
While the therapist may have formulated a view of what is occurring and
could simply offer Sidney an interpretation, there is the danger of setting or perpetuating a norm in which the group waits for the therapist
to address the difficult issues. It is often difficult for group members to
discuss their perceptions of another patient's relationship with the group
therapist. There are many reasons, among which is that such discussions
almost inevitably touch on patients' own wishes for a special connection
with the therapist and their competitive feelings with each other. While
it is difficult to talk about such things, it can also be enormously useful.
One therapeutic intervention is to ask group members what they have
noticed about Sidney's attitude toward and relationship with the therapist. Such an intervention opens up the area of inquiry without disclos-
ing the particulars of the therapist's view so early that members can easily "agree" without thinking about it for themselves. Once again it is
permission-giving—it is saying we can and should talk about these things
in the group—and it therefore should result in an expansion of the boundaries that define appropriate subject matter for the group's exploration.

Of course it puts Sidney on the spot. For this reason, it is important
not only that the therapist be as attuned as soon as possible to how Sidney
is dealing with the material, but also that he or she encourage the other
patients to talk about their views of the therapist's role in the interaction: Is the therapist encouraging it? Does the therapist seem to be allied
with Sidney in a special way? Asking group members to focus on the
therapist diminishes the likelihood of Sidney being scapegoated.

If the therapist believes it to be more propitious to address the issue
directly, it is important to be as nonaccusatory and nonjudgmental as
possible. It is likely that the patient will be defensive anyway, since patients
no more than anyone else like to think of themselves as ingratiating. All
the therapist can do is to try to minimize contributing to whatever defensiveness is elicited. After citing some examples of what has led the therapist to the hypothesis, he or she might say, "Perhaps there is a wish in
you, probably not in your awareness, to please me and get some of the
recognition and gratitude you have never been able to get from your
father."

This is the kind of phenomenon that needs to be repeatedly explored
as long as the patient remains in treatment; the first time it is discussed
it should be construed as laying the groundwork for ongoing exploration. As with many personality traits, ingratiating behavior often comes

so naturally to people (that is, it is so egosyntonic) that it needs to be approached many times in different contexts before therapeutic headway can occur. While it may seem self-destructive to inject dissonance into a pattern that is so useful and gratifying, it is the best service the therapist can provide to patients who are not aware of how they conduct themselves and how their conduct affects others.

The Challenger

On the other side of the coin is the challenging, combative group therapy patient. Such patients can challenge the therapist on any number of fronts: competence, caring, fairness, ground rules, fee policies, and so on. They seem to want or need to fight the therapist at every turn; in fact, sometimes they seem to be challenging the therapist for leadership of the group.

Following is a description of such a group patient.

> Nina, a 29-year-old married female, had recently graduated from a Ph.D. program in clinical psychology, and was the only mental health professional in the group besides the therapist (who was also a clinical psychologist). From the outset of the group, she was unable or unwilling to say much and was clearly struggling with feelings of alienation. Her silence (predictably) drew a lot of attention, and she always was reluctant to say much about what was bothering her. When pressed, she would call into question virtually everything the therapist had done, from how he arranged and composed the group to what he chose to focus on and how he did so. This was all done apologetically and with profuse assurances that she respected the therapist very much and did not want to take issue with him in any way.

Such patients also pose significant countertransference challenges to therapists. Therapists are just as competitive as patients and do not like to be undermined. Particularly when they are insecure, they do not appreciate their competence being challenged. Thus therapists must find a way to deal with their anger with challenging patients in order to maintain a therapeutic stance with them.

If a therapist feels threatened by a patient, the feelings need to be contained and dealt with elsewhere: with a supervisor, with peers, with the therapist's own therapist, or in some other way. The task with the challenging patient is to maintain empathetic attunement and to find a way to explore the interpersonal dynamic while maintaining a positive therapeutic alliance. In order to do this, the therapist cannot feel too threatened; otherwise, anger and defensiveness will overwhelm the therapist's commitment to be helpful.

Once the therapist becomes aware of what is occurring and feels in command of the countertransference, he or she can choose an approach, arrayed on a continuum of directness. Of course it is possible that one or more members will begin talking about their experience of the challenging patient without the therapist needing to say anything. If this does not occur, the therapist can choose a time when feelings about the challenging dynamic seem particularly pregnant and say something as simple as "I wonder what people are feeling now." This kind of intervention redirects the group from whatever the content might be to the unfolding process in the room. If the therapist decides that something more directive is necessary, he or she could say, "I think it would be useful for people to talk about their experience of what seems to be happening between me and Nina." Once again it is important for the therapist to ask patients to comment about themselves as well as the challenger in order to avoid the implication that it must be the patient's pathology that is giving rise to the dynamic.

Alternatively, the therapist can offer an interpretation to the challenging patient either at the time the dynamic begins or at a subsequent point. The challenge is to say something like "You seem to have a need to challenge me at every turn" in a way that is not accusatory. The obvious dilemma is that a therapist can seem (and in fact can actually be) quite defensive when making an interpretation in response to a patient's challenge. For this reason, the substance of the criticism(s) should be dealt with undefensively and *before* the interpretation about the patient's need to challenge the therapist. For instance, if the therapist challenger complains that the therapist seems to favor one of the other patients in the group and the idea seems at least plausible, the therapist could say something like "Your idea that I seem to favor ____ is one I haven't thought of before and one I would like to consider; perhaps you're right." An invitation to explore the patient's need to challenge is more likely to be able to be heard if the therapist has first manifested a genuine and nondefensive willingness to seriously consider the patient's perspective. In essence, it is difficult for the patient not to respond in kind.

The Help-Rejecting Complainer

This is one of the most frustrating kinds of patients to deal with in any modality of treatment. Many patients feel some degree of hopelessness about the prospects for change even as they are presenting themselves to a change agent for the purpose of bringing about change in their lives. Many patients are used to their circumstances in life even if they are unhappy with them, and they are in fact torn between their desire to change and their resistance to change. One of the most prominent ways patients express resistance to change is discounting the possibilities for change they see before them.

Following is an example of how a help-rejecting complainer presents in the group situation.

> Lindy is a 40-year-old single woman who is chronically unhappy but very much used to her circumstances. For instance, she complains about not having found a man but spends most of her time in the group talking about how awful most single men are. She is overweight and unhappy about it, but she has tried every known diet and failed at each one. Even more salient is the fact that her apartment is abominably messy. She reports that there is not a square inch of her floor space that is not covered with old newspapers and magazines or with clothes. The situation is so extreme that she has not had *anyone* in her apartment for over 5 years: men or women, friends, even members of her immediate family. Each and every suggestion or comment made about any of these matters is met with a "Yes, but . . ." response or something equivalent.

Though it sometimes takes a while, it soon becomes clear that such patients are locked into their patterns of living and viewing the world and that they are determined to hold on to their patterns and views (not necessarily consciously) even as they avow that they want to change. Once the therapist sees what is occurring, a therapeutic strategy can be adopted. Since other patients often are extremely frustrated with help-rejecting complainers, a great deal of affect in the group can usually be tapped. A well-functioning group that is working with the dynamics generated in the here-and-now of the group will try hard to find a way to talk about their experience of such patients; in such groups the therapist's primary task is to make sure the feedback remains constructive in nature and that scapegoating is avoided.

However, in many groups participants are not able to find a way to talk about their frustration. Sometimes members are afraid of their own anger and fear that it will emerge in destructive ways if they begin to talk about it. In other instances, members are so fed up with the help-rejecting complainer that they do not want to devote any more group time and energy to the person, even if it means suppressing feelings that it would be relieving to express. In still other instances, members have not put their fingers on what is disturbing to them about their interactions with the help-rejecting complainer; they only know they are frustrated.

The therapist can ask members to consider what they are finding problematic in dealing with the help-rejecting complainer (again being alert to forestalling scapegoating). Alternatively, the therapist can identify what seems to be the prevailing affect: "People who are trying to find

a way to help Lindy seem to be extremely frustrated." However the exploration begins, the therapist wants to get to the point of identifying the
paradox in interacting with such patients, as well as what the group can
do to be helpful. One way a therapist might put this into words is as follows: "The dilemma with Lindy is that she says she wants to change, and
I am sure she means it at one level, but at another level she seems to
have a need to frustrate others' efforts to be of help to her. Our task is
to try to describe this conflict rather than continuing to offer suggestions
to try this or that. If we keep doing that we will just be repeating what
surely happens with Lindy outside the group, and we won't be getting
anywhere."

The tendency for others to offer suggestions will certainly not van-
ish once this is said or even repeated a number of times. However, artic-
ulating the dilemma lays the groundwork for the therapist or other group
members to call a halt to the pattern of suggestions that Lindy meets
with "Yes, but . . ." responses. It forces the help-rejecting complainer to
deal with the group in unfamiliar territory: the old pattern of being
offered suggestions and finding reasons why they will not work has been
replaced. The movement into less familiar territory holds out a possibility for therapeutic movement to occur.

It is important to note that the difficult patient occupies a particular role in a group that can be sustained only with the active participation of the other group members (and sometimes the therapist, as well).
Even when individual patients manifest patterns of behavior that are
clearly well entrenched and used in a wide variety of contexts, the way
others do or do not respond affects what the individual says and does.
In other words, individuals come to take on "group social roles" for which
there is shared responsibility (Mackenzie, 1990).

Once a group therapist understands and has internalized this perspective, he or she has a greater number of options to choose from in
determining how to respond. Although a patient may be addressed
directly, the therapist also might talk about others' roles in what is occurring. The therapist can ask the group why it is choosing to respond
as it is to the difficult patient. This serves an educative function (helping
members appreciate their role in each others' thoughts, feelings, and
behavior) and takes the heat off the individual who is manifesting the
pattern being addressed. Such an approach might shift a group in a way
that frees the individual to interact differently in the group context. While
it is often difficult to know how to address an insecurity being manifested
by a particular individual in a group, the criterion is easy to state: The
therapist should choose the intervention most likely to yield therapeutic
movement for both the individual and the group.

CHALLENGING SITUATIONS

The second section of this chapter will focus on a variety of challenging situations that confront group therapists but are not patient specific. The situations chosen for discussion indicate the range of matters that must be attended to for a group to become, and then remain, a viable working milieu.

Attendance/Punctuality Problems

Whether the importance of regular attendance and punctuality is made clear during the pregroup preparatory phase or later, deviations must be attended to as soon as they begin to appear. Thus, if a group member begins missing sessions, it is important to encourage the other members to express their feelings about it and for the therapist to indicate that he or she is addressing the issue with the patient. Similarly, if one or more patients begin coming late to sessions, it needs to be addressed as a group issue before it becomes a pattern. It is crucial that the therapist begin each session on time no matter how few patients are present; to do otherwise (i.e., to wait until most of the patients have arrived) is to collude in an undermining of the norm the therapist is interested in inculcating. And if the issue is not examined, the therapist can been seen as not being serious; this potential loss of credibility can be fatal to a successful treatment experience.

Of course, to address the issue is not the same as resolving it. In fact, the whole issue of what constitutes resolution is an interesting one. If a person has trouble meeting commitments in his or her day-to-day life, the person can be expected to have similar problems in the group. One of the things patients are told to expect about a group is that they will replicate their familiar interpersonal patterns in the group context. Thus if a person is unreliable in one way or another outside the group, it is *desirable* that he or she replicate the pattern in the group so that it can be examined critically.

Following is a vignette that illustrates how such a behavioral pattern can be worked on in a group context.

> Andrea was on time for the first group session but consistently late thereafter. She had alerted the therapist to the pattern of lateness in her life during their screening interview, so he was prepared for it. When she was 15 minutes late for the second time (the third group session), the therapist asked others to talk about what feelings this engendered in them. He made it clear that he was interested not in people ganging up on Andrea but rather in letting her know the

impact she had on them. Because she was a member who was likable and contributed a lot when she was there, the feedback was not filled with rancor but rather was caring and balanced by many positive feelings.

Not surprisingly, Andrea's pattern continued. Over the course of 12 weeks (it was a time-limited group), she was on time only three times, though she never missed a session. The group got used to her tardiness and seemed to experience it as minimally disruptive. In the course of some sessions, one or more members expressed feelings about her lateness, while in other sessions it was not mentioned at all.

This vignette does not describe a treatment failure. It is rare for chronic, characterologically based patterns to change in 12 weeks. The issue was highlighted for Andrea, and it is not unduly optimistic to hope that she would be able to use her increased awareness to change the pattern over the course of time.

While few group therapists would ask a patient to leave a group for chronic lateness, many would probably terminate a patient who missed sessions regularly. I do not believe this is the best choice under most circumstances. Since patients are usually charged for missed sessions, other patients do not typically feel that the patient is getting away with something without having to pay a price. Also, one patient's irregular attendance does not seem to hold back the group because of the need to fill that patient in concerning what has transpired during sessions at which he or she was not present. My experience is that most groups push ahead with their work and patients who have missed a great deal pick up on as much as they can.

To terminate a patient for living out a life pattern that is one of the reasons, if not the reason, the patient has come into treatment in the first place is usually misguided if the life pattern is not significantly impeding the work of the group. If it is not, the behavior pattern should be viewed as a manifestation of the psychopathology that is the focus of the therapeutic enterprise. It is the job of the therapist and the group as a whole to work with that manifestation in whatever ways the group has at its disposal: to help the person understand it better, to sensitize the person to the impact it has on others, to engender more anxiety and dissonance in the person about the behavior in question, and so on. Such efforts are likely to be much more beneficial to both the offending member and the group than declaring the behavior unacceptable and dismissing the person from the group.

What follows is an example of an attendance problem that was effectively addressed over time.

Irene missed sessions regularly from the beginning of her membership in the group. Typically, she would make either two or three weekly sessions in a month. She never expressed any resistance to paying for missed sessions, and other members' regularity of attendance was unaffected by Irene's pattern. Her explanation was always the same: Her work required her to be out of town. This is a difficult excuse to challenge, since it is assumed to be beyond the individual's control.

However, in this instance, Irene had let the group know that she was a co-owner of her business. After many months of accepting her explanation unquestioningly, different members began to gently challenge her. What was the nature of these trips? What role did she play in scheduling them? At first Irene balked, but members persisted in questioning her, bolstered by the norm that members are accountable to each other, a very strong ethic in this group. Over time Irene was able to acknowledge that some of her trips could be scheduled at different times and that she had been avoiding making this effort because she was afraid of engaging with others and potentially getting close to them (the very issue she had come into group to work on). Her absences eventually diminished, and she began to make headway in lowering the various barriers she had erected to interpersonal involvement.

Of course there may come a point at which it is necessary to ask a frequently absent patient to leave a group. If a patient's pattern of missed sessions is such that the work of the group is impeded, either because the patient is so out of sync with the group that the patient's presence is disruptive or because the absences threaten the norm of regularity of attendance that the therapist has tried to inculcate, termination of the patient from the group may be the wisest course.

Excessive Early Self-Disclosure

Therapists are often concerned about whether group patients will be able to open up and talk meaningfully about themselves. Thus, when a patient brings in material that is emotionally laden, a therapist's initial response is often positive. Such material invariably engages the attention of other members, and focusing on it seems to engender the sense of cohesion all therapists want to see develop in their groups. The therapist hopes that such discussion will lead other members to be similarly self-disclosing.

However, there is danger when patients say more about themselves than they are ready to have others know. Following is an example of how such self-disclosure can be ultimately destructive.

Mitchell, a 47-year-old single male who was being treated in individual therapy by Dr. R, was very sad about his social isolation and was easily moved to tears. Soon after individual treatment began, Dr. R introduced to Mitchell the idea of joining a group. At first Mitchell was resistant, focusing on the fact that he felt so ashamed of much about his past that he could not bear to have others know about it. Dr. R believed he knew what Mitchell was referring to, and he continued to periodically encourage Mitchell to reconsider. Some months later, Mitchell indicated he had come to think it was probably a good idea.

After about 10 minutes of Mitchell's first session, he was predictably asked what he was doing in the group. He replied that there was a great deal of his past that he felt shame about and that he was in individual and group treatment to try to work out these feelings. Once again he was asked a predictable question: Was he prepared to share any specifics? He looked at the therapist momentarily and then launched into a description of his relationship with his estranged brother, which included regular acts of sodomy between them for many years.

Though group members tried to take this revelation in stride, which was the prevailing ethic in the group, they had a difficult time doing so. They were evidently shocked and disgusted by what they heard, though they tried to sound as neutral and nonjudgmental as possible.

The therapist was shocked as well. Though he knew Mitchell was alienated from his brother, the discussions he had had with Mitchell about the relationship had centered on Mitchell's resentment of his brother and feelings of isolation because his brother had been unwilling to have any contact for the last 18 months. However, when the group became engaged in learning more about their history and Mitchell did not recoil from supplying the details that different group members asked about, the therapist felt reassured and did nothing to inhibit the process.

When Mitchell came in for his next scheduled individual appointment, he announced that he would not be returning to the group despite having committed to attending for a minimum of four sessions. Dr. R was tempted to invoke this agreement and use whatever other leverage he could muster, but he restrained himself at first. Mitchell proceeded to tell him that he could not believe how much he had told the group, and, in barely disguised form, he blamed Dr. R for not restraining him. Dr. R tested Mitchell's resolve in a number of ways, and came to see that his decision was irrevocable. He recognized that he had no choice but to report Mitchell's decision to the group and to deal with the fallout (some mixture of anger, guilt, and confusion) that would probably ensue.

This was a particularly difficult case because the therapist was caught by surprise and the information was out before he could do anything about it. Often a patient discusses in individual sessions whether and when to talk about something in a group and/or will broach a topic tentatively in the group session in such a way that the therapist has some time to exercise influence, if necessary.

In general, it is useful for group members to take some time to become comfortable in a group before talking about the most difficult and personal subjects in their lives. Another principle worth keeping in mind is that no patient should get too far ahead of other group members in the level of material being brought into the group. Patients often report feeling comfortable with what they are discussing while in the group, only to become horrified when they look back on what they said and therefore what others now know about them. When this feeling is strong enough, they sometimes conclude that they can never face the other group members again. It is incumbent on therapists to recognize this danger and to exert what leverage they can to dissuade patients from saying too much too soon.

A therapist can intervene in both direct and indirect ways. Sometimes a therapist can redirect a group's attention by commenting on someone else's reaction to what is being said or someone else's interaction with the group member whom the therapist is trying to "save." At other times the therapist needs to be quite direct, either telling the patient that it would be best not to go further with what is being discussed or indicating to the group as a whole that it will not be productive to go further at the present time, that the subject can be returned to when people know each other better. Whatever the approach, the therapist's active effort to short-circuit what is occurring is absolutely imperative.

The "Stuck" Group

One of the most frequent problems therapists struggle with in all modalities of treatment is when the work seems to bog down or get stuck. Though sometimes bogging down takes the form of silence for short or protracted periods of time, more often it takes the form of superficial dialogue. My experience is that this problem is very easy to discern: The telltale sign is that the anxiety level of patients is clearly low.

Bogging down can and does occur in all kinds of therapy groups, but it is especially likely to occur in groups that have a topical focus of some kind. In my own extensive experience in running and supervising groups for patients with genital herpes, patients bring enormous initial energy to telling their stories and to hearing others' tales. After a few sessions, however, the obvious material (feelings toward the person from whom the virus was contracted; experiences of others reacting unfavorably; concerns about whether, when, and how to disclose the information; and so on) has been shared. The group confronts the dilemma of where to go from there. Is the discussion to be limited to matters that directly derive from the condition that brought them together, or is the group going to explore interpersonal issues more generally as they emerge in the here-and-now interaction? The resolution of this issue usually determines whether or not the group will continue to evolve and provide members with opportunities for further growth and development.

The following vignette illustrates the kind of choice point such groups typically reach.

> The group was a time-limited (12 sessions) group for patients with genital herpes. The first two sessions were characterized by energetic discussion of participants' various experiences in dealing with their condition, both internally and in their relationships with others. The therapist did very little as the sense of cohesion developed quickly and naturally.

> At the beginning of the third session, the tenor of the group was decidedly different. Discussion began very slowly, and it was clear that members did not know how to proceed further. Soon Pat, the member who had been most active during the first two sessions, began talking again. She had complained bitterly about the man from whom she believed she had contracted the disease, the variety of men she had met since contracting it, and her parents and various "friends" who had let her down in one way or another. In this session, she began to complain about her boss and coworkers. After about 10 minutes of this, others were fidgeting in their seats but no one was putting their feelings into words.

It was clear to the therapist that other members were experiencing feelings toward Pat (as was he) but that they were unable to articulate these feelings. He thought about asking others to try to express what was on their minds, but he realized that the group's dilemma was that the contract was not clear. Specifically, was it appropriate (i.e., within the bounds of the contract) to express feelings toward each other that emerged as the interaction unfolded, or was the group to restrict its dialogue to the sequelae of having genital herpes? Rather than asking people to plunge into uncharted waters, the therapist indicated that he was aware that the group had been talking only about their experience of having herpes and that it was time to consider whether they wanted to and were prepared to talk about the feelings toward each other that were already beginning to develop and that would undoubtedly continue to emerge as the group evolved. What ensued was a spirited discussion in which some members expressed interest in broadening the acceptable subject matter while others expressed resistance. In this instance, the clear majority favored discussing interpersonal feelings as they emerged, and the therapist articulated the consensus as the understanding with which the group would be conducted.

The decision can be considerably more complicated if the sentiment within the group is more evenly divided. Under such circumstances it is probably best to indicate that the issue remains unresolved and is something the group will need to revisit.

The position the therapist takes in relation to this issue is important. I do not believe the therapist needs to be or should be completely neutral about it. If a therapist believes that the more inclusive contract would best facilitate the group's task, he or she should so indicate and explain the reasons for so believing. Such a straightforward rendering of position should not be confused with pressuring or otherwise attempting to exert undue influence. The therapist usually does have great influence over what a group decides by virtue of being in the role of therapist, and this influence is something to be utilized (albeit judiciously) rather than avoided. If patients genuinely have the room to reach their own conclusion and then live it out, the therapist is justified in trying to persuade them to continue. If a group seems to prefer a contract limited to the discussion of herpes and its sequelae, it is incumbent on the therapist to recognize the emergent consensus and to work in accord with it in good faith.

It is useful to operate on the assumption that a group generally gets stuck because feelings have developed that are not being expressed. The more inclusive contract permits attempting to uncover these feelings and get them out into the open; doing so usually results in a group being able to move forward once again.

The issue of whether a group will be willing and able to deal with conflict among themselves and between themselves and the leader usually emerges early in the life of a group. At a later stage a group can get stuck if it has not worked out whether issues of intimacy can be explored. The following vignette illustrates this issue.

A group that had been meeting for about 3 years began a session with Bob reporting that he and Sara had gone out for a drink and then spent a number of hours talking after the previous week's session. Other members were obviously surprised and began firing questions at both Bob and Sara. When asked what feelings Bob and Sara's action evoked, some members were able to acknowledge feelings of competition and envy. However, discussion of such feelings did not progress very far, and soon the group grew quiet. Efforts to discuss other subject matter also did not get very far. It became clear to the therapist that the group was stuck, and he was convinced it was related to the news with which Bob had begun the group. As the therapist thought about it, he realized this was the first time a group member had alluded to feelings of attraction to another group member, either directly or indirectly. He did not know how to address this at first, and he ultimately decided to say what he had thought about it.

This intervention opened the floodgates. What followed was weeks of discussion of some of the positive feelings that had developed between and among group members over the years. Some of the work was very painful, and feelings of shame about these feelings, especially when they contained a sexual component, were prominent. It became clear to members how long they had avoided these feelings and how much more difficult it was to talk about attraction and intimacy than it was to talk about conflict and aggression.

Obviously, things do not always progress so easily; this was a well-functioning group that needed very little help in moving into a new (and difficult) area of exploration. When an intervention of the sort made in the vignette elicits little if any material, the therapist does well to plant the seeds for future work by saying something like "Perhaps you can give some thought to what kinds of feelings of attraction to others in the group you might be harboring and which ones you might be able to divulge at some point in our work." Similar words of encouragement can be expressed in subsequent sessions as opportunities present themselves. Often such efforts bear fruit weeks or months after they are begun.

Scapegoating

Scapegoating is one of the most common problems that emerge in therapy groups and also one of the most dangerous; it is therefore one of the most important challenges a group therapist faces. What is obvious is that the individual being scapegoated is at risk for being damaged, perhaps seriously. What is less obvious is that the group as a whole is threatened, because a scapegoating process that is not well managed can lead everyone in the group to feel unsafe. This in turn can lead to group members limiting their participation in the group or perhaps even leaving the group in order to avoid being scapegoated themselves.

Following is an example of a group situation that was ripe for a scapegoating dynamic to unfold.

Peter, a 32-year-old single man, entered an ongoing therapy group of young adults. He was a painfully obsessive man whose presentation from the outset made it plain that there was a real possibility that a scapegoating process could ensue. Some time during his first session he was asked why he had come to group, and his response was extremely convoluted and unclear. Similarly, when he commented on others' situations, he was extremely long-winded and difficult to follow. As a result, the pace of the group's work slowed down dramatically, and others' frustration with him began to build very quickly.

The therapist was alert to Peter's danger from the outset. At first she asked people to give feedback to Peter about his presentation. While it may seem tantamount to inviting other members to scapegoat him, it was a good initial strategy for two reasons: It is almost always better to encourage people to get feelings out into the open rather than letting the feelings simmer and ferment because they cannot be expressed, and it was a test to see whether Peter could respond to the feedback he received about how much frustration he was eliciting.

In this instance, it became clear that Peter's style was not easily influenced. Though he was clearly affected emotionally by the feedback, he did not respond by withdrawing; rather, he continued to try to contribute to the group in a quasimechanical way.

The second strategy the group therapist attempted was to redirect the attention of the group onto those who were most vociferous about their frustration with Peter. While a great deal of their frustration could be accounted for by how objectively difficult Peter's presentation was, it was nevertheless therapeutically significant that some group members responded with as much venom as they did. One patient discovered how narcissistically injuring it was for her to be derailed when she was in the middle of relating something important to her; Peter reminded another of his younger brother, whose physical disability had been extremely costly to him during his formative years.

While this strategy reaped some useful therapeutic fruit, the difficulty with Peter did not diminish. The therapist struggled to confront something that seemed increasingly obvious: She had erred in bringing Peter into the group. He simply did not have the ability to engage in the level of psychological work the group was doing. After struggling for a few weeks to acknowledge this to herself, she did so and made the painful decision to remove Peter from the group.

The therapist called Peter and arranged for an individual session, during which she acknowledged the obvious: Peter was not able to engage with the group at the level at which it was functioning. Though Peter must have been injured by this acknowledgment, he did not manifest any palpable response to the news, though he did refuse the therapist's invitation to return to the group for a final session. In consultation with his individual therapist, the group therapist referred Peter to a more appropriate group.

At the following group session the therapist announced that she had removed Peter from the group and indicated that Peter had declined her invitation to return for a last session. She felt that the group needed an explanation, and after briefly describing her thinking process, she emphasized that it was her mistake. The therapist met efforts to talk about how frustrating it was for members to deal with Peter with suggestions that group members were avoiding talking about their feelings about the therapist having erred. There was no question that group members' confidence in the therapist was affected by her error, and it took persistent exploration of the negative transferential responses this episode elicited over a number of sessions to work this through.

Following is an example of an incipient scapegoating process that was successfully resolved within the group.

Tina, a 36-year-old white single female, entered the group at a time when a number of group members were opposed to a new member being added. There were seven members in the group, and four of them expressed reservations about a new member being added at that time. The group therapist paid close attention to what group members had to say, but she ultimately decided to bring Tina in because she felt that Tina could benefit from a group experience.

During Tina's first session she behaved in a way that was utterly predictable to the group therapist. She was most eager to talk about herself and not really attentive to the concerns that other members expressed. The therapist knew that group members would not respond favorably to this, especially since they were resistant to a new member coming in, so she realized that Tina was at risk. As members began expressing their annoyance with Tina, the therapist closely monitored how she seemed to be responding. Because she believed that part of the group's response was brought about by Tina's interpersonal style, she attempted to help her understand what people were responding to. However, as the feedback continued and intensified, she took a different tack.

Specifically, the therapist suggested that some of the intensity of feeling that was being directed at Tina was actually meant for her. She pointed out that bringing Tina into the group was her decision, and that it was clear that people were distressed that she had done so in the face of strongly felt opposition to the addition of a new member. When members insisted that their feelings toward Tina were legitimate and not simply displaced from the therapist, the therapist did not disagree; she persistently refocused the group on their anger about her decision. As a result, Tina was able to integrate herself into the group and she was able to hear and work with the feedback about her egocentrism.

This vignette illustrates the important point that anger directed toward another group member is often a displacement of feelings toward the leader that cannot be expressed or at times even acknowledged. This displacement does not negate the legitimacy of the feelings as they are expressed. Rather, it suggests multiple determinants for the feelings; the therapist often has to choose which of the determinants to focus on. If a new patient in a group is getting a lot of negative feedback, it is often a good idea for the therapist to emphasize the transferential component, as new members need to be protected from getting too much negative feedback too quickly. If they are not protected, they are at high risk for premature termination.

Overt Conflict between Members

In some ways group therapists welcome overt conflict between group members: It can lead to a great deal of interpersonal learning for the parties involved in the conflict, as well as for the others in the group, and is certainly enlivening and engaging for everyone in the room. The following vignette describes a conflict that was resolved in a conventional fashion.

Francine talked about her conflict with her son Ivan, who was 25, from the beginning of her tenure in the group. She obviously did not know how to relate to Ivan in a constructive way, and she periodically responded to him in a very authoritarian way, which she had many opportunities to do because Ivan still lived with her. Francine met group members' suggestions of alternative strategies with "Yes, but . . ." responses, and things continued to deteriorate between her and her son.

Billy, who was 32, found himself growing more and more hostile toward Francine. It soon became clear that he identified closely with Ivan (whom he had never met), largely because his relationship with his parents was in many ways parallel to Ivan's with Francine. As Billy became more strident toward Francine, the therapist pointed out the parallel between the two family situations. While it seemed transparently obvious to the therapist, it came as something of a surprise to Billy. Thereafter, other patients periodically asked Billy to talk about his family rather than to take out his frustrations on Francine. The net result was that Billy came to focus more and more on his family legacy, both in group and in individual therapy, and the nonproductive tension between Billy and Francine largely dissipated.

Interpretive measures do not always work when conflict emerges in a group, and some conflicts can be threatening to the group's continued existence. One such type of conflict is the fight that is so explosive that others are frightened and no longer feel safe in the group. Another is the protracted and unresolved struggle between two members, which can lead to hopelessness and despair in the parties directly involved and in other members (and the therapist) as well.

Following is a vignette that is an amalgamation of these two forms of potentially destructive conflicts and that required a risky intervention before the group could move on.

Michael had been a member of a long-term group for about 18 months, and Al had joined the group about 6 weeks prior to the session described. Michael was quite long-winded and members had periodically expressed their frustration with him. Al too had done so on a few occasions.

At the beginning of this session, Al came in distressed about his job situation and began to describe some of the details. Very quickly, however, Michael began talking about his history of job failures. While his tale seemed relevant at first, the connection with Al's concern seemed more and more remote as Michael continued to talk. Other members were getting increasingly uncomfortable, but no one interrupted him for quite some time.

Finally Al exploded, and he did so in a way that was very frightening to others. He became apoplectic: His eyes bulged, his veins popped out of his neck, and he screamed at the top of his lungs. Furthermore, what he said was vicious: He berated Michael in the most disdainful way as a worthless human being. The therapist thought there was a good chance that Al was going to physically assault Michael, and he was sure that others thought there was an even greater danger of it. He was prepared to physically restrain Al if it was necessary.

While he did not have to, it became clear that the group was traumatized by what occurred. Members were much more cautious and tentative than they had been heretofore, and this persisted over the course of a number of weeks. Therapist-initiated efforts to discuss what had transpired led to some acknowledgment that it was frightening but to no diminution in patients' obvious cautiousness.

As the therapist thought about it, he came to see that what had occurred had changed members' primary tasks: They were primarily focused on avoiding trouble rather than bringing in material to be explored. Put simply, the group was no longer experienced as a safe milieu. His efforts to address the problem at this level elicited acknowledgment that people were feeling unsafe, but there was no appreciable change in the atmosphere that pervaded the group. In the weeks following the initial explosion, Al had a series of smaller explosions; he continued to find Michael enraging, he was beginning to find others only slightly less so, and his unleashed anger grew.

The therapist felt that the continued existence of the group was in jeopardy, and he knew he had to do what he could to bring about a change as quickly as possible. He was seeing Al in individual therapy, and he talked with him about his concerns about the group. He did not dispute Al's contentions that his feelings were shared by everyone in the group and that he was fulfilling the agreement as it was presented to him (namely, to report the feelings he experienced as they emerged in the here-and-now of the group). The therapist explained that he drew a distinction between the constructive expression of anger, which contains a desire to help the other learn something, and the destructive expression of anger, in which hatred and the wish to injure are the underlying sentiments. The therapist asked Al to contain his feelings when they seemed to fall into the latter category.

The therapist was uncomfortable about this strategy. It was incontrovertible that Michael was a source of frustration for everyone, and it was true that Al was fulfilling the treatment contract as it had been prescribed to him. Nevertheless, and somewhat to his surprise, Al seemed to understand the distinction the therapist was drawing and the rationale for asking him to monitor himself. His outbursts disappeared immediately, though he and others continued to express their sentiments to Michael when they became frustrated with him. Though it took some time, the feeling of safety returned to the group and it carried on with its work.

When a conflict in a group becomes too explosive or goes on too long without resolution, it can be discouraging if not damaging for everyone involved. It is incumbent on the therapist to find some way out of the morass. Of course, at first the therapist does whatever is possible to help patients explore the nature of the conflict that has emerged and what each party can learn from it. If the conflict persists in a way that seems to be bogging down the group's work over a protracted period of time, the therapist may as a last resort suggest that, because the group does not seem able to find a way out of the struggle, it would be best for everyone to think of it as an unresolved problem that cannot be usefully discussed any further at this time.

Extra-Group Socializing

Practitioners usually address the issue of what forms of interaction might occur between group participants outside group sessions during the preparatory (pregroup) phase. But early attention to the issue certainly does not mean that it will not emerge as the group evolves; it does mean that the therapist needs to think the issue through before beginning to meet with prospective group patients.

In thinking about the issue, the therapist must acknowledge certain realities. First, some interaction between patients outside the context of the group is inevitable: Patients usually gather in a waiting room before the group begins, and they all leave the therapist's office at the same time. With respect to time immediately before and after group sessions, then, the issue is not so much whether patients will interact at all, but rather whether agreed-on guidelines will govern their interactions. Specifically, a therapist might ask patients not to discuss matters pertaining to the group during such interactions. Alternatively, the understanding might be that if discussions pertaining to the group do occur, they will be reported to the group.

Second, the therapist must decide what his or her position is on the guideline. A therapist can *recommend* or *require* that a particular guideline be followed. I strongly prefer the former. First, requirements tend to invite more acting out than recommendations. Also, recommendations are characteristic of adult-to-adult communication, involving the judgment of the person to whom the recommendation is being made, while requirements are characteristic of parent-to-child interactions. In this sense, recommendations are more consistent with the overall goal of treatment, which is to strengthen the autonomous functioning capacity of the patient.

Another factor to be considered is the functional level of the patients in a group. Generally speaking, the higher-functioning the patients, the less interaction between sessions is desirable. With lower-functioning patients who generally lack support in their everyday lives, connections with other group members can come to constitute a support system. Since support groups are often long-term, this support system can meet important needs for a substantial period of time; in addition, members may learn some basic social skills that they can bring to their interactions with others.

The rationale for discouraging (or attempting to prohibit) contact between higher-functioning patients outside the context of group sessions is that outside contact dissipates the dynamics of the group, which are best explored during the group's work time. Of course, almost any guideline (or requirement) is periodically broken; the challenge is to make such breaches therapeutically useful.

The following is a vignette about a high-functioning group that had an understanding that patients were not to have contact between sessions.

At the beginning of the session Bob indicated sheepishly that he had something he wanted to talk about. After glancing at Carol a number of times, he reported that he and Carol had had dinner after last week's session.

This news caused quite a stir in the group. It was the first violation of the extra-group socializing guideline, and it was a substantial one. However, group members did not talk about the violation per se; rather, they were intensely curious about what had occurred.

As Bob and then Carol gave their respective versions, it became clear that Carol was the one who was most disappointed with how things had gone. Whereas Bob was uncertain when asked if he would like to spend more social time with Carol, Carol was unequivocally not interested. Though she seemed somewhat concerned about hurting his feelings, she made it clear that she did not find Bob at all appealing. Carol's expression of her feelings was embarrassing for Bob and uncomfortable for the other group members.

This episode presented a great challenge to the therapist. Her first decision was to steer clear of the collusion of Bob and Carol in acting out against her and the exploration of others' feelings about this. She knew this issue would need to be addressed eventually, but it was not the first order of business. What seemed necessary first was to bring into the group what had been acted out: that is, to get Bob and Carol to describe their respective experiences of their time together and to have other members voice their reactions.

The struggle for the therapist was averting the possibility of grave narcissistic injury to Bob in response to the particular material that emerged and at the same time acknowledging Carol's right to her experience and to express her feelings about it. The therapist permitted Carol her freedom and also took pains to indicate to Bob that she was aware of how difficult Carol's material might be for him to hear; and Bob seemed to feel supported by her as well as a number of the other members of the group.

The exploration of the acting out by Bob and Carol and what it represented for the group as a whole took place over the next several sessions. Both Bob and Carol were able to acknowledge the thrill they experienced in getting together surreptitiously, and others spoke of the vicarious excitement they felt as well. Feelings of jealousy and fantasies about romantic and sexual liaisons were also acknowledged by a number of group members. The therapist emphasized that it was clear that Bob and Carol were expressing sentiments and desires that many group members were feeling in one form or other.

After the group looked at what had happened between Bob and

Carol, as well as the feelings it evoked in others, the therapist felt the need to reinforce the guideline discouraging substantial extra-group socializing. She did not want to sound reprimanding in doing so as a parent–child relationship between therapist and patient discourages the atmosphere of safety that is most conducive to open-ended exploration. So she specifically stated that she did not feel upset with Bob and Carol in particular; she acknowledged that the episode had, in fact, triggered a great deal of useful work for many group members. At the same time, she reiterated her recommendation, and she reiterated her rationale as well: Such contacts outside group can result in subgrouping that is very difficult to discuss and thus often avoided, and such subgrouping can lead to feelings of competition and envy that can destroy a group. At the same time, she indicated that if such contacts were ever to occur again, she would like the people involved to handle it just as Bob and Carol had.

Premature Termination

Therapists do well to discuss termination during the preparatory phase of group treatment. It is useful to instill the notion that ending treatment should be discussed in the group (though the ultimate decision is the individual's to make) and that there should be an ending phase to the treatment experience rather than an abrupt departure from it. While such efforts at norm-setting can be helpful and are certainly worth doing, they do not eliminate the phenomenon of abrupt unilateral terminations.

Such terminations occur at all phases in the treatment process. This section takes up two examples of this phenomenon, one occurring early in a patient's treatment experience and the other occurring at a much later point. The early one follows.

> Don entered an ongoing group and was asked to make a six-session initial commitment, which he readily did. He took an active role from the outset, which was surprising to the therapist and at first pleasing to her. However, the nature of the contributions Don made were almost uniformly off-putting to the other members of the group. He responded very concretely to the dilemmas others described and gave advice that was premature, filled with clichés, and not at all helpful. In the second session members began expressing their chagrin about this, and though it was quite muted, Don found it very difficult. Unsurprisingly, he called before the third session and said he would not be returning.
>
> The therapist responded with immediate relief when she got the message, and thought the group would as well. When she announced it in the group, however, the expressions of relief she expected were

rapidly followed by expressions of dissatisfaction with her for bringing Don into the group. This led to weeks of productive though difficult (at least for the therapist) work about long-held feelings within many group members about how the therapist was conducting the group. She did not make contact with Don, largely because she knew he was in long-term treatment with a colleague of hers; she did of course speak with his therapist about her perspective concerning what had occurred.

The later premature termination occurred under very different circumstances.

Sheila had been in the group for 18 months. About 6 weeks before she left the group she began a relationship with a man named John. While people in the group were pleased for her, they also expressed concern about how quickly she was moving ahead in the relationship. They kept reminding her that she did not know John well yet and told her she sounded as if she were making premature assumptions about both him and their future together. She communicated her decision to leave the group by leaving the therapist a message indicating that things had gone awry with John and that she was too distraught to continue treatment.

The therapist tried to contact Sheila before the next scheduled session, but she was unsuccessful. When she told the group about what Sheila had decided, some group members were primarily angry with Sheila for her hasty decision about the group, while others focused on their sympathy for the disappointment she must be experiencing.

The therapist emerged from the session with a determination to set up an individual session with Sheila. She knew that Sheila had just begun individual treatment with another therapist, but she had no idea whether she was continuing it. She had not yet spoken with the other therapist, but she felt that the longevity of her relationship with Sheila justified an intervention on her part. She wanted to provide whatever help she could to Sheila in her effort to work through the loss of John and to talk with her about the possibility of continuing in group treatment.

She decided to wait a few days before attempting to reach Sheila, and during this time Sheila called. The therapist suggested an individual session, making clear over the telephone what her dual agenda was. Sheila agreed to the idea and indicated that she had stopped her individual treatment on the same day she had quit the group. The therapist ended up seeing Sheila for two individual sessions, at the conclusion of which Sheila decided to resume group treatment.

The therapist decided to pursue Sheila for a number of reasons: the length of their relationship and the positive therapeutic alliance she felt they had; the absence of a well-established individual therapy relationship; and her conviction that Sheila's decision was impulsive and ill-advised. She made sure to clearly identify her point of view but to avoid twisting Sheila's arm and to focus primarily on the crisis in Sheila's life rather than what she was going to do about group treatment.

Diminishing Group Size

Therapists wrestle with the issue of optimal group size both in the process of beginning a group and at points in the life of a group when the number of members diminishes. How many patients are enough to start a group? How many members are required to continue a group?

While different practitioners undoubtedly have different numerical answers to these questions, certain factors need to be kept in mind. First, perfect attendance at every session cannot be expected, no matter how compliant the patients in a group might be. Thus, if a therapist feels that four patients is an absolute minimum for a viable group session, just four members in a group is not sufficient. Second, it can be debilitating to patients' morale (not to mention the morale of the therapist) to continually be concerned about whether enough patients will be in attendance for a group session to be viable. The third factor, however, sometimes runs into direct conflict with the second: To delay beginning a group that patients have been waiting for or to suspend a group until more participants can be found risks losing the members the group already has. Some patients may opt to join another group, some may choose another form of treatment, and some may give up the idea of treatment altogether. This is why decisions about what to do with groups that have a marginal number of participants can be so difficult.

Following is an example of such a dilemma.

An ongoing group had been functioning with only five patients for quite some time. While the therapist wanted to add new members to the group, he did not feel it was urgent because the five group members attended very consistently and seemed to be working well together.

Returning to his office about an hour before a session was scheduled to begin, the therapist got a message from Vicki: She had decided to leave the group and would not be there that evening or thereafter. Though Vicki had been struggling with some issues during the last few weeks, the therapist was caught completely by surprise. He decided to try to reach her to ask her to come to the group to discuss her thinking, but he got her answering machine when he called. Given the definitiveness of her message, he thought it was unlikely that she could be prevailed upon to return in the future.

This not only left the group with only four members, but it also left it with just one female. Both Diana and Vicki had made it plain that having another female in the group was crucial for them, and the therapist held the belief that it is imperative to have at least two men and two women in a group for it to be viable.

The therapist reported Vicki's message to the group at the outset of the next session. After the patients expressed their feelings about her decision as well as their speculations about why she had made it, the question of the status of the group was raised. The three male members expressed the wish to continue working with four members until the therapist found one or more suitable additions, but Diana was much more equivocal: Part of her wanted to continue, but she feared being the only female in the room.

The therapist indicated that he would think about what people had said, as well as do his own thinking about the issue, and let them know the following week what he had decided. The next session he announced that unless he found a suitable female to join the group within the next 3 weeks, he would suspend the group until he identified such an individual. Members seemed to accept this plan. Since no one emerged over the course of the next 3 weeks, the group was suspended; 2 months later it resumed with two new patients, one male and one female.

This is one of the many areas of group therapy on which there is no real consensus among experienced practitioners. Some believe that the group should continue to meet for a period of time even when the number of patients is marginal, arguing that the continuity of meetings is crucial in creating a secure and predictable therapeutic frame. Others believe that it is too debilitating for patients and therapist alike to wonder from week to week whether an adequate number of patients will show up for a viable group session. There is even substantial disagreement about what constitutes an adequate number of members for a viable session; some believe that two is enough, while others believe that four or five are minimally acceptable.

In the situation described here, the therapist decided that it was not viable to continue with only one female patient. He invited members to be in touch with him during the hiatus, and he touched base with them every 2–3 weeks to keep them posted about the status of the group. When the group resumed, the work proceeded in an exciting fashion, so the therapist felt that the wisdom of his decision had been confirmed.

CONCLUSION

The difficult patients and challenging situations discussed in this chapter are by no means an exhaustive representation of the problems that confront group therapists. Group patients bring the full range of their psychopathology to treatment; in addition, the interpersonal, subgroup, and group-as-a-whole dynamics that are played out in the group treatment setting result in an enormous range of problematic situations over the course of time. While each patient or situation has its own flavor, can any generalizations be drawn about how therapists should respond to them?

I believe that therapists need to be proactive rather than laissez faire in addressing problems—if not immediately, then sooner rather than later. Sometimes the therapist facilitates the exploration of the issue in question by the group members, while at other times the therapist must take the lead.

Certainly, each circumstance must be responded to in terms of the characteristics of the group at that moment: where the group is in its development, what kinds of resources exist within the group to take on the issue, what kind of threat (if any) the patient or situation poses to the group's healthy functioning and continued existence, and so on. But the generalization about proactivity should govern our thinking as group therapists, mostly because problems that are not addressed usually do not spontaneously resolve themselves; rather, they tend to fester and become worse over time. There is nothing more debilitating for a group than to be unable to make headway with a problem, particularly one which either starts as or becomes time-consuming. The resulting helplessness and hopelessness are the antithesis of the tone and attitude that facilitate movement and change. It is part of the job of therapists to recognize this threat and to use all the tools in their arsenal to come to grips with the issue in one way or other. In this way the therapists fulfill the primary role responsibility of their job: to do whatever is possible to make the group experience a productive one for participants.

REFERENCES

American Psychiatric Association. (1987). *Diagnostic and statistical manual of mental disorders* (3rd ed., rev.) Washington, DC: Author.

MacKenzie, K. R. (1990). *Introduction to time-limited group psychotherapy*. Washington, DC: American Psychiatric Press.

Yalom, I. D. (1985). *The theory and practice of group psychotherapy* (3rd ed.). New York: Basic Books.

• SIX •

SELECTION
OF GROUP
INTERVENTION

Judith Schoenholtz-Read

The selection of a group intervention for a client depends on the relationship between the potential client and the factors specific to the group being considered. What do you, as a clinician, need to understand when you refer a client to a group? What are some of the client factors that need to be identified when matching the client with the appropriate group? Given the range of group interventions now available, such as short-term outpatient groups, residential addiction group programs, long-term psychodynamic groups, specialized groups for the sexually abused, and 12-step groups for alcoholics and others, what are the group factors that need to be identified?

We now know that many different kinds of people benefit from groups (Lieberman, 1990). They include a wide range of patients, from the severely mentally ill to those with addictive disorders or problems related to abuse, and nonpatients, such as family caregivers and bereaved parents. Surprisingly, the effectiveness of group therapy is not widely known. Few are aware that outcomes of group psychotherapy have been demonstrated to be as effective as outcomes of individual therapy (Whiston & Sexton, 1993).

Although evidence shows that all types of groups are helpful, we as clinicians must rely on our clinical experience to guide us in matching the potential group member with the most appropriate group. Matching a client with a group is a complex task for all therapists and is not unlike choosing appropriate individual therapy for a client: Given the range of individual interventions, how does a therapist choose the most effective form of therapy? There is little research to guide either the individual or the group therapist. Psychotherapy researcher Lester Luborsky and colleagues (1993) characterize the problem: "Finding good matches of type of patient and type of treatment is a recurrent dream of psychotherapy researchers; the satisfaction of the wish in waking life has mostly been elusive" (p. 546). Although the core elements of psychotherapy that influence outcome have not been definitively identified, most clinicians accept that common processes related to the interactive elements between the client and the therapist are shared by all therapies (Whiston & Sexton, 1993).

In group psychotherapy, the relationship between the leader and the group member seems to be less important than the group members' relationships with each other as a group. Group cohesion, or how well the group is perceived as functioning together, is seen as one of the best predictors of outcomes (Dies, 1993). Although there is no well-established system for predicting the positive outcome of group interventions with particular types of patient problems, there are ways to identify a wide variety of patient factors and relate them to different group interventions.

In the process of evaluating patients for group psychotherapy, we learn about their presenting problem and investigate their history of interpersonal relationships. To be successful in making the appropriate referral to group treatment, there needs to be a good fit between how the patient's problems are conceptualized by each group approach, their etiology and the therapeutic change process. Each type of group intervention differs in its understanding of the patient's problem and the method required for therapeutic change. In this chapter, the patient/client factors we focus on are (1) the severity of the patient/client's presenting problem or level of functioning, (2) the patient/client's motivation for change, and (3) the patient/client's expectations and goals for therapy. The group interventions we focus on are (1) inpatient and partial hospitalization groups for acute or chronic patients, (2) outpatient groups for all types of patients, and (3) "other-than-therapy" groups for a variety of participants.

Assessing the severity of the client's presenting problem can be done by measuring the client's psychological health–sickness (PHS). Psychological health–sickness refers to general adjustment, ego functioning, personality integration, emotional stability, and overall mental health—a global condition that has been a consistent predictor of positive psychotherapy outcomes. PHS can be measured by the Health–Sickness Rating Scale (HSRS), the Minnesota Multiphasic Personality Inventory (MMPI) Global Severity Measure, and the Global Assessment Scale (GAS), which is part of the Axis V diagnosis in the *Diagnostic and Statistical Manual of Mental Disorders*, third edition, revised (DSM III-R) (Luborsky et al., 1993).

The most extensive research has been done on the HSRS. This scale uses 30 case examples to derive 8 100-point scales that include a global scale and 7 criterion scales. The criterion scale items are the need for protection as opposed to level of autonomy, the severity of symptoms, the level of discomfort, and environmental effects. The interviewer matches the patient to the comparable case in the 30 examples. Studies utilizing the scale indicate that the diagnosis does not often correspond to psychological health or sickness. Major diagnoses differ widely in level of psychiatric severity, for example, the diagnosis of psychoses ranges in severity from 0 to 50.

The GAS is an adaptation of the HSRS and has been incorporated into the DSM III-R Axis V. The clinician rates a 90-point scale to evaluate functioning on a variety of dimensions both at present and during the past year. Low scores (from 1 to 50) indicate severe impairment: The client may be dangerous to self and/or have severe and disabling symptoms. Moderate scores (in the 60 range) suggest ability to function at home and work with moderate symptoms. Mild distress (above 70) indicates mild symptoms and only minor impairment at work, at home, or in social functioning.

The Global Severity Measure on the MMPI is a self report measure which summarizes the most elevated clinical scales to determine the level of distress. Overall, research strongly demonstrates that the degree of severity of the client's problem together with diagnosis, rather than diagnosis alone, is predictive of outcome (see Luborsky et al., 1993).

Broadly speaking, patients' problems demand certain responses from the clinician. Patients whose problems are severe or whose mental health is very poor—for example, the suicidal and acutely psychotic patient—need protection in the form of hospitalization. Patients who have mild to moderate psychological health problems can benefit from weekly outpatient group treatment. Others fall somewhere in between and may require partial hospitalization or some combination of individual and group treatment. Some patients may have moderate to serious problems and be unmotivated for psychotherapy, yet they may be willing to address certain aspects of their problems and can be prepared for group therapy during a pretherapy orientation or a psychoeducational group approach. Patients who have completed the formal therapeutic task and need help to maintain the changes they have made respond to a wide range of support groups, 12-step and self-help groups, which I refer to as "other-than-psychotherapy" groups.

In this chapter, group interventions will be described in a systematic way to help the clinician match patient with intervention. In each section, types of group intervention, each intervention's theoretical understanding of the patient's problems, and the therapeutic change process will be discussed. The approach of the chapter is summarized in Table 6.1.

COMMON CHARACTERISTICS OF HELPING GROUPS

Although the differences among the variety of group interventions are many, we need to recognize the important similarities among groups—including "other-than-psychotherapy" groups—without regard to theoretical orientation or setting. All small "helping" groups develop the common purpose of working together toward specific therapeutic goals. When we account for the therapeutic properties of the helping group, we give value to the powerful factors that are mobilized when a group of individuals gathers to help one another.

Lieberman (1990) characterizes the helping group as a "small, face-to-face, interactive unit" (p. 4) of people in distress that is led by professionals or nonprofessionals. Members come together because they are in need. In the group, members are expected to share their distress. This shared suffering, Lieberman believes, is the key element in the development of group cohesiveness, which in turn allows group members to take risks and express emotions not usually revealed. Each group forms a closed system with its own set of rules and norms. The members perceive that they are different from others outside. In a sense, the group becomes like a family; it bonds together in a special setting that provides support, acceptance, and the normalization of experiences. One of the

TABLE 6.1. Overview of Types of Groups

Psychotherapy groups for severe problems	Psychotherapy groups for mild to moderate problems	"Other-than-psychotherapy" groups
Inpatient group programs	Outpatient group treatment	Support groups: General and specialized
Acute psychiatric unit	Short-term general groups	
Chronic psychiatric unit	Short-term specialized groups	Peer-led support groups
Drug/Alcohol treatment	Long-term general groups	12-step groups
	Addictive disorder groups	Professional support groups
Partial hospitalization	Medical problem groups	
Traditional day hospital	Crisis center groups	
Innovative day treatment		
Halfway house/residential treatment		
Psychiatric medication groups		

powerful group forces that promotes change is the members' desire for group acceptance, which leads to conformity to group rules and behaviors. How to talk and what to talk about are all part of the group culture. The pressure to change in the direction valued by the group is a powerful motivator. The potential threat of exclusion influences members who desire the group's appreciation, praise, and "consensual validation."

Groups that encourage a wide range of behaviors and experiences are usually more successful. All groups typically support and have specific techniques to induce the expression of strong feelings. The group atmosphere reduces the need for the conventional controls over emotions, and it values the expression of strong affect, such as anger, hurt, fear, and sadness. One of the mechanisms of change common to all groups occurs when members are able to compare their experiences and responses. By observing and modeling others, group members can learn new ways to perceive, think, and feel about their problems.

For example, in peer self-help groups such as Alcoholics Anonymous (AA), group members are expected to share their common problem and demonstrate commitment to one another. The ideology requires belief in the uniqueness of the group members and the group program. An assumption that there is no other available help bonds members. Cognitive restructuring takes place through an organized ideology that defines the origins of the problem and the processes for change through a prescribed set of behaviors, or steps.

Similarly, therapy groups, whether they are long-term or short-term, psychodynamic or cognitive-behavioral, have their own set of assumptions about the etiology of the patients' disorders and beliefs about what cures. These assumptions and beliefs emerge directly and indirectly through the structuring of group norms, leadership behaviors, and group processes. For example, in a description of a short-term intervention for victims of post-traumatic stress disorder (PTSD), Scrignar (1990) indicates how the principles of the group program are related to assumptions about PTSD. Five themes are emphasized: misconceptions about the disorder, uncontrollable thoughts, avoidance, increased arousal, and numbing of general responsiveness. The structured group treatment addresses the assumptions about the etiology of PTSD and includes education, cognitive restructuring, relaxation training, exposure treatment, assertiveness training and anger reduction, family relationships, and problem solving. Scrignar's work clearly illustrates how the assumptions about etiology and cure are closely tied to beliefs or theoretical understanding. He specifically states that the psychodynamic conceptualizations of PTSD are not helpful and constructs his treatment approach within a cognitive-behavioral framework. This example highlights how the clinician's belief system regarding etiology and change forms the framework for group intervention. In self-help peer groups, these principles are manifested as powerful ideologies or program ideals and requirements; in psychotherapy groups these principles are theory-based.

Even though the 12-step and cognitive-behavioral groups are structurally different, they are similar in their effort to develop group cohesion, a necessary element for any well-functioning group. Yalom (1985) characterizes cohesion as "absolutely integral" to effective group development. He describes it as the attractiveness members have for one another and the group. A cohesive group is one in which members accept and support each other in the change process. It can be seen as parallel to the patient–therapist relationship in individual therapy. As well, cohesiveness includes group-formed conditions of safety and acceptance that make self-disclosure possible. Research supports the importance of developing close and positive bonds among group members as significantly related to productive therapeutic work (Dies, 1993).

The social environment created by the interpersonal interactions of the members of a group becomes the powerful vehicle for therapeutic change. Group psychotherapies use the group members' interactions as a main focus for the therapeutic work. The "other-than-psychotherapy" groups tend to view group members' interactions as a global factor supporting the individual's work. Vinogradov and Yalom (1989) illustrate the perspective that stresses the importance of interpersonal relationships as a therapeutic factor. Indeed, it is the basic theoretical principle of their view of psychopathology. For them, psychological distress is the result of interpersonal distortions originating in childhood experiences. When the group addresses the individual's maladaptive interpersonal reactions and assumptions that have been recapitulated in the group, change can take place through "corrective emotional experience."

The interpersonal processes in the psychotherapy group support the possibility of a corrective emotional experience. First, the group needs to be experienced as a safe place to express deep feelings and differences; then, when there is honest feedback that permits reality testing, the group behaves like a social microcosm. Over time, group members show their historic and problematic behaviors to each other. New interpersonal learning occurs through a process carefully outlined by Vinogradov and Yalom.

1. Members show their interpersonal pathology to one another.
2. Members give feedback about each other's behavior and "blind spots."
3. Members share reactions to one another's feedback.
4. Individual members have a clearer picture of their behavior as seen by others.

5. Individual members learn how their behavior affects others, and this helps clarify their distortions.
6. A responsibility for changing behavior develops.
7. With the acceptance of responsibility for change comes the realization that one can change.
8. The depth of change is related to the degree that affectively laden events are expressed in this process.

We can see that Yalom emphasizes the importance of interpersonal learning and responsibility; it is the "cardinal mechanism for change" in long-term, unstructured groups. Research supports his view that interpersonal feedback and self-disclosure are positive factors for change (Dies, 1993). Even in groups that do not explore the group members' interactions as the major group focus, the interpersonal context is still seen as the environment that supports change (Tables 6.2 and 6.3). The more general factors that promote change include "hope" inspired by work-

TABLE 6.2. Differences between Psychotherapy Groups and "Other-than-Psychotherapy" Groups

Psychotherapy groups	"Other-than-psychotherapy" groups
Participant expectations	Participant expectations
Desires professional framework	Willing to participate without profes- guidance
Accepts group contact as part of the therapeutic process	Needs or desires support rather than more intensive exploration of behavior
Willing to examine behavior patterns through group and individual interactions	Attendance and payment may be voluntary or flexible
Therapist and context factors	Leader and context factors
Professionally trained leaders	Nonprofessional or peer-led
Contract to work under certain conditions	No formal group contract; emphasis informal commitment
Clear therapeutic goals and techniques	Less clearly defined member/leader group boundaries
Theoretically based interventions	Emphasis on social support and pragmatic interventions rather than theoretically based interventions
Use of group as a social microcosm	Little attention to group process as a whole or interpersonal interactions
Specific admissions criteria and diagnoses	Admission based on self-identification of a problem or defining issue
Group members' compatibility a selection factor	All members accepted who are willing to participate
Development and enforcement of group norms	Variable enforcement of norms

TABLE 6.3. Importance of Therapeutic Factors in Psychotherapy Groups and Other Groups

Therapeutic factors	Psychotherapy groups	"Other-than-psychotherapy" groups
Instillation of hope	Moderate to high[a]	High
Universality	High	High
Imparting information	Low to moderate	High
Altruism	High	High
Development of social-izing techniques	Low to high	Low to moderate
Imitative behavior	Moderate	Moderate to high
Catharsis	High[b]	Moderate
Corrective recapitulation of family group	Moderate to high	Low
Existential factors	Moderate to high	Low to moderate
Group cohesiveness	Moderate to high	High
Interpersonal learning	High[b]	Low
Corrective emotional experience	Moderate to high	Low
Group as a social micro-cosm	Moderate to high	Low
Self-understanding	High[b]	Low

Note. Information from Vinogradov and Yalom (1989).
[a]Inpatient groups
[b]Long-term outpatient groups

ing for a common goal; "universality," which occurs when group members recognize that others have similar distress; and "altruism," which results when group members help one another (Yalom, 1985).

In the interpersonal world of different psychotherapy groups, the curative factors are consistently identified by group members as related to being with others. Yet group members often notice, over the course of the group's development, that different factors seem to be more important at different times. In the early phases of all groups, members are preoccupied with creating a safe environment and building cohesion. In the later phases of groups, members who give and receive both positive and negative interpersonal feedback and thereby contribute to the quality of the group experience tend to benefit most from the group (Kivlighan, 1985).

Now that we have reviewed some of the powerful elements that are active in all helping groups, we will discuss a systematic way to identify for patients/clients the most appropriate group intervention. The three sections that follow present patients with severe problems in need of hospitalization or partial hospitalization, outpatients with mild to moderate problems who can benefit from a group within the broad range of outpatient groups, and clients who can be supported by "other-than-psychotherapy" groups. Each section identifies the specific forms of appropriate group interventions and how to evaluate the best match for your client by becoming familiar with the goals of the different interventions and the approaches they utilize.

GROUP INTERVENTIONS FOR PATIENTS WITH SEVERE PROBLEMS

Patients with severe problems include people who are actively suicidal and/or acutely psychotic, severely anorexic, in need of drug or alcohol detoxification and treatment, or in severe interpersonal crises. When these patients can no longer be maintained in the community, the clinician may decide that inpatient treatment is required for their protection, assessment, and support. Group treatments can be found in acute psychiatric inpatient units and in specialized treatment programs such as programs for alcoholics, drug addicts, or people with eating disorders.

Group programs in acute psychiatric inpatient units are highly variable in quality, nevertheless, Leszcz and colleagues (1985) found that patients who participate in inpatient groups very frequently experienced benefits. As the influence of managed care providers increases, the full impact on inpatient treatment programs remains to be seen; however, in efforts to cut costs, it is likely that the duration of inpatient stays will be decreased. Kibel (1993) describes the confusion in inpatient treatment programs. In general, acute psychiatric treatment units have treatment programs that incorporate group activities, but the integration of the group offerings into the overall treatment program varies considerably. It is important to be familiar with a unit's program and philosophy to determine if the program is the most efficacious for a patient.

Rice and Rutan (1981) identify criteria (the "outside contract") that provide a systematic way for the referring therapist to evaluate the quality of an inpatient group psychotherapy program. Although it may be difficult for an outsider to determine if the criteria are met, they are worth consideration.

- Are the goals of the group program integrated into the overall treatment program?
- Is group therapy an equal part of the treatment system?
- Are the patients expected to participate in the groups as fully as in the other activities?
- Does the group treatment begin immediately after admission?
- Is communication between the staff and the group therapists adequate to provide a good exchange of information about the patients' experiences in group therapy?

- Does an obvious interdependence among the staff reflect mutual rather than competitive goals?

General Types of Inpatient Groups

Inpatient groups must accommodate many patients who would ordinarily be excluded from outpatient groups. In addition, inpatient group programs need to respond to the range of severe patient problems, the differences in patient motivation, and the various durations of patients' stays in the hospital. To deal with the variability in patients' level of functioning and length of stay, many programs have adopted the "level" approach. Following are descriptions of four group approaches that take into account the patients' level of functioning.

Yalom's level approach (1983) provides all patients in the unit a group program. Patients participate in two groups. One is a "team group," which includes 6 to 10 patients across diagnoses. It is led by an interdisciplinary staff team and meets daily. The other is a "level" group composed of higher-functioning patients or lower-functioning patients. The level groups meet three to four times a week rather than daily; not all patients are expected to participate, but those who do must attend each session. Both the team and the level groups share basic norms of confidentiality, time boundaries, and appropriate behavioral limits. In the lower-functioning level group, the more distressed and impaired patients focus on their responses to one another, and the leader is actively involved. The higher-functioning group uses interpersonal focus to examine the group members' reactions to one another through a series of exercises and activities facilitated by a here-and-now approach. The focus in all the groups is on adjustment to the unit, the instillation of hope, and the importance of interpersonal reactions of others as a way to improve one's own behavior. Yalom's approach attempts to provide a coherent structure with carefully defined norms to respond to the diversity of tensions, agendas, and needs in the acute unit.

Brabender's short-term model (1985) is designed for higher-functioning patients who can keep the rules, tolerate some emotional discomfort without becoming self-destructive, have some ability to separate fantasy from reality, and have an ability to control emotions and listen to others, as well as a willingness to commit to a two-week hospital stay. Brabender's approach attempts to deal with the competing ward demands by structuring the group composition and norms to insure stability. She argues that the structured, closed group permits the members to experience greater cohesiveness through the group's developmental phases. Unlike most acute inpatient groups, Brabender requires all patients to participate in eight sessions and to enter and leave the group on the same day. In addition, not all patients are placed in the group, even though they might benefit; selection is based on the balance of patient resources. The therapeutic focus is on psychodynamics; the therapist interprets the underlying conflicts in the group as a whole and relates the symptomatology to unconscious themes according to the group's developmental stage.

Kanas's short-term approach (1990) utilizes a homogeneous group to treat hospitalized schizophrenic patients. Kanas has found that schizophrenics can benefit from the interpersonal environment of the therapy group during acute episodes. Hallucinating and delusionary patients who are willing to be in a group and talk with others do better than those who are withdrawn or isolated. Although other approaches suggest that schizophrenics can be mixed with other patients, Kanas proposes that there is more cohesion when the group members have similar presenting problems and symptoms. The goal of the group is to get the patients to interact with each other and begin to solve problems, a goal that is difficult to achieve when the patients are experiencing loose associations and active hallucinations. Kanas suggests that in the homogeneous group, the therapist can use techniques more appropriate for the schizophrenic patient. For example, there is evidence that techniques that encourage self-disclosure and expression of affect can be harmful for schizophrenic patients. What is more helpful is focusing on improving relationships with people, which might include spending less time in their rooms or finding ways to cope with their hallucinations. Group members give hope and help to one another. Kanas's groups meet three to five times a week for 45- to 60-minute sessions.

Kibel's psychodynamic approach (1993) considers the patient's level of functioning but emphasizes the importance of the patient's internal processes as reflected in relationships with the therapist and other group members. Kibel's first goal is to help patients understand their experience in the unit. Other benefits of the group include improved relationships with others, more positive self-esteem, better management of aggression, an improved relationship with staff, and an improved sense of reality. Kibel suggests separating patients who are predominantly psychotic from those with character disorders or affective illnesses.

Who may not benefit from inpatient groups? Kibel (1993) suggests the following guidelines for the exclusion of patients:

- Cognitively impaired patients such as those with possible organic brain syndromes
- Severely regressed patients who cannot express their simplest needs
- Patients who cannot tolerate even low external stimulation

- Patients who have little impulse control so that the group safety may be threatened
- Patients who are self-injurious and need close supervision
- Patients who justifiably elicit serious anxiety (as distinguished from countertransference in the therapist)

Who benefits from inpatient groups? The Leszcz, Yalom, and Norden (1985) study of patients' responses to level groups suggests overall satisfaction with inpatient group psychotherapy but marked differences among types of patients. The more regressed, lower-functioning patients preferred the compulsory and less intense team group; the higher-functioning patients were often frustrated by the team group and preferred the more intensive, structured, and verbal level group. The Leszcz, Yalom, and Norden study suggests the importance of fit between the patient's expectations and the group's goals. For example, those who did not like the level group wanted advice and did not value self-understanding or self-expression. These patients' goals were more compatible with the team group, which was more concrete and gave advice. Conversely, those who did not like the team group wanted more self-understanding.

Specialized Inpatient Groups

Specialized groups for patients with eating disorders and patients with severe alcohol and drug addictions are beneficial for patients who are required by their physical condition or their own motivation to seek inpatient treatment. Some treatment units are now available to patients with dual diagnoses and other more complex problems.

There are certain advantages to a homogeneous inpatient approach for certain patients. Typically, addiction units treat addictive disorders and utilize, to varying degrees, a therapeutic community model that has strict group norms and requires abstinence from drugs and alcohol. On the average, specialized inpatient treatment programs are 28 days, a short time to convince the patients that they must change. And many patients must be convinced: They were brought to the hospital by a concerned relative or friend and themselves are unmotivated. Flores (1993) argues that the "art of treating addiction is to overcome the enormous denial and resistance" (p. 436) that may be expressed passively or with open rebellion. If the therapist understands that in the early stage of treatment (1) the addicted patient's judgment and behavior are cognitively impaired by the addiction and (2) the patient will fail to relate interpersonal problems with substance abuse, the therapist will be prepared to use persuasion to get the patient into group treatment, where all the therapeutic group forces can be brought to bear to help patients recognize that they alone are responsible for abstaining from alcohol or substance abuse. However, it is only in the second stage of treatment, when some degree of abstinence is gained, that psychotherapy can begin to be effective. Then group members confront the relationship between their dependence on substances and their difficulties with close relationships and life's demands.

Inpatient addiction programs often integrate a 12-step approach, like that of AA, with psychotherapeutic treatment. AA provides patients with a supportive peer group that can encourage maintaining abstinent behavior after discharge. A more careful discussion of combining group psychotherapy with "other-than-psychotherapy" groups is presented at the end of the chapter.

Partial Hospitalization Programs

Partial hospitalization or day programs have begun to increase and will continue to develop with efforts to control full inpatient costs. Many patients need more than weekly individual treatment yet do not need to be hospitalized or can be maintained outside the hospital with close observation and intervention. These patients range from those with chronic mental illness such as schizophrenia and severe affective and anxiety disorders to those with eating disorders and some personality disorders.

Many day programs suffer from the problems found in inpatient units: patients' problems are diverse and the time commitment is variable. By trying to serve all types of patients in the same setting, these programs often fail to use their potential. However, many day treatment programs are undervalued by the hospitals that offer the treatment. The programs may suffer from staff demoralization and underutilization. Some problems occur when the programs try to accept all types of patients and combine disorganized or lower-functioning patients with more organized and higher-functioning patients. One the other hand, when the programs make some effort to separate the psychotic and/or chronic patient from the neurotic and/or personality disordered, the possibility of powerful group treatment becomes a reality.

Traditional day treatment has most commonly been care for the chronically mentally ill. Most often patients whose psychological health–sickness is considered poor, such as patients with schizophrenia, bipolar disorder, or major depressive disorders and some personality disorders, fall into the category of patients who may need to have a daily supportive environment. Treatment goals for acute or chronic patients who suffer from serious interpersonal deficits need to be realistic and focus on how to improve the patients' quality of life. The day hospital group interventions are most appropriately organized to stress survival and social skills. Brier and Strauss (1984) suggest that the group treatment needs to reflect the stage of the patient's illness. In the initial recovery stage, patients indicate that interventions that include ventilation, social approval, reality testing, material support, and problem solving are most useful; for those in the "rebuilding stage," symptom monitoring, interrelating, and motivation are particularly valuable.

The primary task of day programs may vary from transition to the community to maintenance. The programs are usually grounded in some form of therapeutic community model that immediately engages patients in an interactive group process. Group activities vary from verbal therapy and art and music to vocational training. Day treatment programs often include family members in special family groups as a way to help the patient deal with family problems and develop better skills to cope with stressful family situations. The comprehensive approach to day treatment can be advantageous for many patients. Careful matching of treatment goals with patients' PHS must be done when making a referral to day treatment.

GROUP INTERVENTIONS FOR PATIENTS WITH MODERATE PROBLEMS

Patients with moderate problems live and work in their communities yet benefit from group psychotherapy. They include people with symptoms of depression or anxiety and those with eating and life-style problems, as well as those who have longstanding problems relating to others. People with characterological problems and with alcohol and drug dependence are in this group. Group psychotherapies have been found to be effective with people who have these problems as well as with more chronically mentally ill people who are able to live in their communities.

A number of factors influence the selection of an outpatient group intervention.

Patient factors that should influence the choice of outpatient group intervention include material and psychological factors. The material factors are the patients' insurance benefits and limitations and the time the patient has available for treatment. Psychological factors are the severity of the patient's problem and the patient's history of interpersonal relationships and patterns. The psychological factors may influence the intensity of treatment the patient can tolerate. A patient who is isolated and has a history of difficult interpersonal relationships may be more appropriate for a short-term group whose goals are less ambitious than intensive short-term or long-term groups. The patient's psychological mindedness and motivation for change are critical factors to evaluate in addition to the patient's expectations and goals. A patient who wants to attend group therapy to meet other people to socialize with may not be appropriate for a group; yet if the patient can accept that the purpose of the group is to learn about one's behaviors that lead to interpersonal difficulties, then the group referral may meet the individual's needs.

Therapist factors are treatment orientation, assessment of the patient, and bias toward specific forms of intervention. The flexibility of the therapist and openness to different approaches naturally affect the group selection. In some cases, the therapist refers clients to other therapists who can make a better match.

Contextual factors are the setting and duration of the group and the homogeneity or heterogeneity of group members' problems, family histories, genders, and/or cultural backgrounds.

One of the major dilemmas when making outpatient referrals is how to conceptualize the patient's main problem in order to refer the patient to either a long-term or a short-term group, a homogeneous or heterogeneous group, and so on. The dilemma of how to assess the patient's needs is particularly salient in the following kind of situation.

Suppose a patient has a history of trauma: childhood sexual or physical abuse, for example. Is it best to refer such a patient to a short-term group for trauma survivors or to a longer-term heterogeneous group? In the longer-term heterogeneous group, the therapeutic emphasis will be less on the trauma itself and more on the personality organization and interpersonal dynamics as consequences of the trauma. A short-term group for sexual abuse survivors will focus on the disclosure, telling the story of the trauma, encouraging others to tell their stories, and how to respond to others to prevent retraumatization.

To make an appropriate referral, the therapist must carefully assess how the patient identifies, describes, and conceptualizes his or her problem. The therapist can help the patient choose an appropriate group in a pretherapy training experience. Pretherapy sessions include didactic information and structured interactions that can help inform the patient about group processes and goals, teach the patient how to interact in a group, and explore the patient's level of commitment and activity. In general, evidence shows that pretherapy training improves attendance, helps to determine psychological mindedness, and influences dropouts (Salvendy, 1993).

Short-Term Outpatient Groups

Short-term group psychotherapy offers outpatient treatment to a wide range of patients and can be classified broadly to include groups that are heterogeneous but vary according to theoretical orientation and those that are organized homogeneously according to diagnosis, presenting problem, life themes/issues, gender, and/or developmental phase (Table 6.4). Most short-term groups meet for between 8 and 20 sessions and are closed to new members. The groups comprise from 4 to 15 members. It is important to consider patient expectations when making a referral to a time-limited group.

MacKenzie (1993) has identified the basic patient, therapist, and contextual factors of brief therapy groups.

Patient factors

• Careful assessment is needed to exclude patients who may not benefit from an active approach.
• A contract is developed identifying specific and limited therapeutic goals.

Therapist factors

• The therapist is active and maintains the group focus on the specific group and individual goals.
• The therapist focuses on the interrelationship between what members learn in the group and how they apply it outside the group.
• The therapist expects the patient's to initiate therapeutic tasks and encourages group members to do so.

Contextual factors

• The time limit increases the expectation that the therapeutic work will proceed quickly and be applied to life situations outside the group.
• Mobilization of outside group resources is encouraged to support the positive changes.
• It is expected that the change process will continue after therapy terminates and that there is a limit to what can be achieved in the group.

Heterogeneous Short-Term Groups

A short-term group with a specific theoretical orientation may include patients with different kinds of problems. The patients are chosen according to level of psychological health and fit with the theoretical orientation.

One of the most important short-term group models has been developed from cognitive-behavioral principles. This kind of group tends to include a psychoeducational approach and offers structured activities to

TABLE 6.4. Examples of Types of Short-Term Groups

Theoretical	Diagnosis	Theme	Gender

Cognitive-
  behavioral
Interpersonal
Psychodynamic
TA-Gestalt
	Anxiety
	Chronic pain
	Depression
	Eating disorder
	Post-traumatic
	  stress
		Adult children of
		  alcoholics
		AIDS patients
		Bereaved
		College freshmen
		Victims of child
		  sexual abuse
			Women
			  Battered women
			  Sexually abused women
			
			Men
			  Alcoholics
			  Batterers
			  Drug abusers

facilitate change according to a specific understanding of the cognitive etiology of patients' maladaptive behaviors. Exercises help patients understand how their thinking about events, their underlying assumptions about themselves, and their beliefs about the outcomes of specific activities may be unfounded. A method for correcting faulty thinking provides the material for the group work. The approach helps group members recognize their faulty thoughts and unrealistic expectations. They practice new ways of talking to others and thinking about things. Some of the groups offer relaxation training and training in assertiveness skills. Such techniques are designed to help the group member feel more in control by restructuring beliefs about the world. In these groups, there is little emphasis on catharsis and interpersonal interactions, which makes this approach suitable for patients with high anxiety and depression who will respond to a collaborative and structured therapy.

Innovative Short-Term Heterogeneous Groups

Another type of short-term heterogeneous group is the intervention that combines a variety of approaches. As the pressure to find more efficient mental health treatment models increases, more short-term group treatments are integrating the best elements of day treatment, therapeutic community, brief psychotherapy, and family systems.

In most mental health systems, a large number of demoralized patients tend to drift from therapist to therapist without significant improvement; they need more intensive treatment than individual and/or weekly group therapy can offer. These patients do not need hospitalization, but traditional day care is not intensive enough. They have some neurotic symptoms and personality problems, typically complain of depression, anxiety, obsessional behaviors, and eating disorders, and often have a history of alcoholism and/or drug abuse. These patients have severely damaged self-esteem, and they often have family histories of physical and sexual abuse. They need an intensive intervention program that provides powerful tools for restructuring self-defeating interpersonal patterns.

The Integrated Psychotherapy Group model (Knobloch & Knobloch, 1979) is an example of a program that can treat such patients. The approach is based on a theoretical integration of contemporary psychotherapies, combining aspects of psychoanalytic, cognitive-behavioral, social learning, and systems theories with therapeutic approaches like psychodrama, guided fantasy, and expressive therapies (art, music, and dance). The intervention also is an adaptation of the therapeutic community model and therefore permits treatment of a large group of patients at one time.

Some of the essential features of the Integrated Psychotherapy Group model are (1) structuring the group to model daily life activities—work tasks, sports and "family" groupings—so that members' social networks, interaction patterns, and life styles are evoked and can be studied; (2) using the group setting to evoke the maladaptive patterns, observing them, and exploring new interpersonal solutions; (3) applying indirect methods, such as psychodrama, and direct methods that involve participation of significant others in special weekly family group sessions; (4) mobilizing group forces through the use of a patient committee that collaborates with the staff to enforce the group's norms; (5) creating a "surplus reality" through fantasy games, weekly plays, ceremonies, and expressive therapies; and (6) developing an interdisciplinary therapy team to unify group strategies, review patient interactions and progress, and support one another and the group norms. Through a variety of structural innovations, the therapeutic environment maximizes the potential of the group for therapeutic change (Lazerson, 1984, 1986).

Specialized programs of this kind require clearly defined patient selection criteria. For example, patients who have a history of psychosis or are actively suicidal probably should be excluded; so should those who need to be on psychotropic medications and those who have serious physical impediments that make them unable to participate in a sports program. In addition, patients who have serious addictions to alcohol and drugs and are not at a point where they are capable of abstinence should be excluded. Inclusion can be determined by the patient's commitment to attend the program daily for 6 weeks, abstinence from street drugs, writing a daily journal, attendance at three weekly aftercare sessions, willingness to keep group confidentiality, as well as the willingness of "significant others" (partners, friends, parents, siblings, bosses, coworkers) to participate. Pretherapy training is used to orient all prospective patients to the community norms. The norms are enforced by a patient committee that is elected weekly and is supported by the staff;

the committee can use specific methods to support the individual group members as they progress toward their therapeutic goals (Lazerson, 1986).

Intensive psychotherapy groups of this kind have broad application and can provide effective treatment for patients, particularly those with personality disorders, who tend to be difficult to treat in weekly individual or group interventions. Clear boundaries and norms are set and enforced by the patient community and the community can be powerfully mobilized to support individual and group therapeutic goals.

Homogeneous Short-Term Groups

One of the important ways to decide whether a patient needs heterogeneous intervention or a specialized group is to evaluate the patient's need to identify with a specific problem or issue and the need for symptom relief. Homogeneous groups can be based on members' disorder(s), gender, previous childhood experiences, adult developmental issues, addictions, and so on. Some patients can be motivated to seek therapy by identifying with others who have similar problems; others benefit from a specific therapeutic orientation. For the most part, heterogeneous short-term groups include members with a broad range of problems and tend to utilize the group process, particularly interpersonal interactions. Homogeneous groups tend to develop cohesion quickly through identification with common problems and may be less intensive than heterogeneous groups (Klein, 1985).

It is not unusual to find that specific theoretical orientations are used in specific patient groups. For example, in a therapy group for herpes patients, Drob and Bernard (1986) separately applied cognitive and psychodynamic approaches. In their loss groups, Piper, McCallum, and Azim (1993) utilized psychodynamic techniques, as did Beckett and Rutan (1990) in their work with AIDS patients.

AIDS patients illustrate some of the issues when considering homogeneous groups. Their unique problems make them ideal to treat in a homogeneous group. The AIDS patient is facing impending death, and the certainty of death often makes relationships with healthy persons difficult; the problems of healthy persons can seem trivial to the dying patient. Beckett and Rutan suggest that in a homogeneous group of AIDS patients, the members perceive their own uniqueness, and their ability to support one another is strengthened. Patients terminally ill in other ways and even patients who have had other unique life experiences can also benefit from a homogeneous group.

Another form of homogeneity that might influence referral decisions is gender. Increasingly, short-term groups for mild to moderate

problems are offered along gender lines. What are some of the considerations in referring a patient to a single-gender group as opposed to a
mixed-gender group? First, of course, is whether separate-gender groups
and mixed-gender groups are equally effective. Although there is no clear
empirical evidence (Huston, 1986), clinical evidence shows that for some
women an all-women's group can be more therapeutic than a mixed-
gender group.

What are the relative advantages of the all-woman's group? Some
are developed with the clear goal of attending to gender issues from a
feminist perspective. The all-women's group that is constructed to attend
to women's roles within the social, political, and historical context can
be therapeutic for women with certain presenting problems and particular life experiences. There is some consensus that women who have been
sexually or physically abused or are socially isolated from other women
benefit from an all-women's group. Specifically, women's groups provide a safe place to join other women, to end isolation, and to explore
women's stereotypic roles and behaviors. In the all-women's group
women feel safer to tell their stories and through mutual support to
empower one another. The group becomes a place where the responses
to hierarchy and power relations with men, as well as the development
of empathy toward oneself and new models of strength, can occur. Oakley
(1992) describes the "women's group space" as providing a unique level
of safety that promotes openness and bonding that members may not
have experienced before.

Spending time with other women gives women the opportunity to
relive the adolescent phase of development in which girls try to create a
separate and safe world but often fail to do so. Recent research on adolescent development supports the view that women can prosper in their
own space (Gilligan et al., 1981). Girls who attend all-girls schools seem
to have a stronger sense of self than other girls. This provides a strong
argument that a women's group can offer an empowering and a cogni-
tive-emotional corrective experience for many women.

Some women's groups are homogeneous not only in gender but also
in theme. Herman and Schatzow (1984) and others have described groups
for women with a history of sexual abuse. These women may feel very
unsafe exposing their secret in a mixed-gender group and may find a
women's group the first safe place to begin to deal with the experience
and consequence of abuse. But other women clients with similar symptoms, such as anxiety or depression, may benefit from a mixed-gender
group. The client factors that need to be considered when matching a
female client with a women's or a mixed group are the client's developmental history, history of interpersonal relations (particularly with men),
and present motivation for group treatment.

When should a man be referred to a men's group? Some men's groups have been developed to focus on specific destructive behaviors, such as battering, alcohol abuse, or drug abuse, while others are for men who have problems with intimacy. In general men are more reluctant than women to enter psychotherapy. Krugman and Osherson (1993) attribute this reluctance to men's stereotypic adherence to an image of male stoicism and invulnerability. Often motivated for treatment by a crisis, such as marital breakdown or job loss, men still cling to a mask of competence and control. Initially, many men view the psychotherapy group as a social club, a sports team, or a work group so that they can feel familiar in it. With carefully regulated exposure, men can be opened up to risk attention to their emotional needs and to learn new interpersonal skills.

The mixed-gender group obviously has the advantage of permitting men and women to explore gender-related differences, such as emotional expressiveness, attachment (dependence, independence, and interdependence), power, and competition, as well as stereotypes that tend to maintain distance and misunderstanding between the genders. Skillful leadership is required in such groups. When gender differences and stereotypic responses are left unattended, they can only reinforce disempowerment and pathological responses in female and male clients; yet when the mixed group confronts gender-related behaviors, attitudes, and values, profound shifts in intimacy, self-awareness, and social stereotypes can occur (Lazerson & Zilbach, 1993).

Long-Term Heterogeneous Outpatient Groups

Long-term groups are groups that meet regularly for more than a year. Although one of the most common forms of longer-term group is the group with an interpersonal orientation, this type will be addressed only briefly since the principles were described in the section on characteristics of helping groups. The focus of this section will be on the longer-term group run according to psychodynamic principles.

Alonso and Swiller (1993) clarify some of the elements that characterize psychodynamic groups:

1. *Vital enactment of the characterological dilemmas of the members.* In the group the members experience their effect on others; they learn from others and discern how their perceptions are distorted. They can experiment with new behaviors while they share in the universality of human suffering.
2. *Exposure and resolution of shameful secrets.* By sharing important secrets, patients experience the fears of others. The empathetic group environment enhances the individual's well-being.

3. *Support for the universality of the member's wishes, fears, and distress.*
   The group provides unique support for one another's pain and
   suffering as well as understanding of the more negative human
   emotions.
4. *Reintegration of the split-off parts of the self.* Features of the group
   members' unconscious aspects of themselves emerge in the
   group, are mirrored by others, are understood as human, then
   are forgiven and dealt with.

In order to create the atmosphere for the dynamic healing process
to occur, all the different psychodynamic orientations include some of
the following dimensions.

- *The goals* are to restructure the personality through a process that
  relies on analysis of the internal or unconscious aspects of self, as
  well as the internal object relations as they are projected onto other
  group members. How the process occurs varies according to each
  orientation and how each conceptualizes the patient's internal and
  external dynamics.
- *The therapeutic environment* is viewed as critical; the setting is made
  safe by clear boundaries, tolerance, and support that are modeled
  by the therapist and encouraged by other group members.
- *Dynamic concepts* such as transference, countertransference, projection, resistance, introjection, and projective identification are
  used as part of the therapeutic process and are understood to be
  the vehicles of change.
- *The role of the therapist* is to provide the safe environment and to
  clarify, confront, and interpret group interactions. (Interactions
  vary according to different dynamic orientations, as do timing and
  level of activity.) Attention is paid to group processes as they occur
  at the structural and the individual level.

The work of Kibel (1992) describes how change occurs in a long-
term dynamic group. The prerequisite for change is the development of
a safe environment. Each individual's particular ways of obstructing the
development of a trusting relationship with the group must be modified
and eventually dissolved for therapeutic progress to occur. When a safe
environment is established, the "maladaptive habitual responses, assumptions, and interactions" (p. 55) can be studied and changed through the
mechanisms of imitation, identification, and internalization.

Imitative learning occurs when members observe successful members share emotions and difficulties and adopt similar behaviors. This

enhances the desire to belong, makes the group attractive, and increases cohesion.

Identification is the process in which group members take on aspects of other group members and recognize the possibility of altering their perceptions and affects. However, identification can function to enhance either change or resistance. Peer identification develops as members tell their stories and reactions to events in and outside the group. Identifications are feelings of similarity and attraction that are extended to universalization when members recognize that they are not alone. A circular process occurs that continually enhances the identifications. For example, a male group member states that he learned to be a better father as he listened to a female member's stories of her maltreatment by her father. The male patient recognized his caring for his daughter and was able to express it more openly as he identified with the female group member's need for love. Rutan and Stone (1993) note that imitation and identification are so powerful that they can explain how even inactive group members may benefit from the group.

Internalization is the intrapsychic level of change and occurs, as Kibel emphasizes, through a shift in psychic structures. As patients interact through identification and imitation, the therapist clarifies and interprets behaviors in the here-and-now. Members gain understanding about their reactions, assumptions, and values. The outcome is an integration of affect and object relationships that diminishes inner conflict.

Who benefits from psychodynamic long-term heterogeneous groups? In general, the kinds of patients who can benefit include a broad range. It is clearer to therapists who will not benefit (Baker & Baker, 1993). These are patients who are skeptical and need to be pushed to join a group; actively suicidal patients; people who are extremely defensive and highly narcissistic; and people who have prior relationships with group members outside the group. Increasingly, dynamic therapies are working with more severe character pathology. However, the person who is sociopathic, is explosive, or has a brain dysfunction, as well as the person in severe crisis who may demand a great deal of attention and the person who will not agree to the basic contract (Rutan & Stone, 1993), are not good candidates.

Although I have focused on psychodynamic group psychotherapy to illustrate the relationship among the patient and group factors that provides for a good therapeutic fit for long-term groups, I would like to mention some of the other forms of long-term groups that are available and some of the advantages for particular types of patients. Groups with an interpersonal orientation utilize the patients' interactions with one another in the here-and-now in a directive and structured way (Yalom, 1985). The focus is less on the internal restructuring of object relations and the manifestations of unconscious needs and conflicts than on the behavioral manifestations of interpersonal strategies as they are played out in the group. Many of the theoretical constructs mentioned in connection with psychodynamic groups are not the main considerations of the interpersonal therapist. This approach may be particularly valuable for patients who cannot tolerate the regression that may occur in more psychodynamic groups when the therapist may be relatively quiet and noninteractive. Patients who have specific interpersonal problems, such as those resulting from divorce, impaired relationships with children or coworkers, and so on, and who need a more directive approach, may respond to interpersonal orientation.

Transactional analysis, Gestalt, and psychodrama are other forms of long-term group therapies and have developed different conceptualizations of psychopathology and active techniques to deal with internal and interpersonal conflicts. These approaches emphasize the mobilization of strong affect and catharsis as a way to change patients' relationships to the unconscious aspects of themselves. Patients actually identify different parts of themselves through directive techniques. The active interventions facilitate the patients' awareness of conflicting needs and desires. The corrective emotional experience occurs when patients enact split-off parts of themselves or replay, by role taking, a new solution to a problem. For example, in TA or Gestalt therapy, a patient may play herself and her critical mother. In the corrective experience, the patient tells the mother how hurt and angry she has been because of particular childhood experiences. The mother accepts the criticism instead of putting the patient down. In psychodrama, the patient chooses another group member to play the role of the mother and the childhood scene is replayed with a different solution. Both role playing and psychodrama use active interventions and move quickly to heighten affective states that are seen to underlie unresolved interpersonal situations and influence the patient's present behavior. These approaches vary in how much they utilize the group process. They have been criticized for neglecting the responses of the group as a whole and for working with the individual within the group. I no longer consider this a fair criticism of these approaches (Kepner, 1987; Kipper, 1992). These approaches are particularly useful for patients who tend to intellectualize and seem out of touch with their affect and disconnected from their experiential world.

GROUP INTERVENTIONS FOR MODERATE TO MILD PROBLEMS

In addition to psychotherapy groups, there is a wide array of "other-than-psychotherapy" self-help groups (Table 6.5). In California alone, over

TABLE 6.5. Examples of "Other-than-Psychotherapy" Groups

Support	Self-help	12-step	Psychoeducational
Abuse survivors	ANAD (anorexia and	Abanon	Cardiac recovery
Addictions	bulimia)	(Abortion)	Communications
Adoption	Compassionate	Addicts Anonymous	skills
AIDS	Friends	Alanon	Coping with pain
Alzheimer's	Healing Hearts	Alcoholics Anonymous	Meditation
Arthritis	Parents Without	Cocaine Anonymous	Parenting
Battered women	Partners	Codependents Anonymous	Postpartum recovery
Binet (bisexuals)	THEOS (They Help	Debtors Anonymous	Self-improvement
Cancer survivors	Each Other	Depressives Anonymous	Stepparenting
Coping with pain	Spiritually)	Families Anonymous	
Dyslexia		Living Positive	
Eating disorders		Narcotics Anonymous	
Gay/Lesbian		Overeaters Anonymous	
Parents of adoptive		Parents Anonymous	
children		Sex Addicts anonymous	
Parents of teens		Workaholics anonymous	
Quit smoking			
Women/Men			

3000 self-help groups include the well-known 12-step groups for various specific problems and support groups of many different kinds. Lieberman (1993) argues against generalizing about self-help groups. He stresses that the stereotype of the leaderless and boundariless group has created a negative attitude toward self-help groups that have as a positive strength adaptability to meet members' needs. The wide variety of "other-than-therapy" groups can provide help to many who have mild problems due to a life crisis such as the death of a family member or a recent health or situational trauma; to people who are at a similar life stage; or to those in need of special skills to improve their mental health. In addition, many of these groups can provide ongoing support for those in the maintenance phase of therapy.

Leadership in the "other-than-psychotherapy" groups includes nonprofessionals who are trained by their organization as well as untrained peers; the leaders and members are powerfully drawn together by ideas that enable them to create a unique experience. Hope, understanding, and care permeate many groups' primary values; the groups provide social support; and they offer a cognitive restructuring by endorsing a particular conceptualization about how the group members' suffering comes out (Lieberman, 1993).

Self-help and 12-step programs can be attractive to individuals who are willing to identify a specific problem and want some help but do not want to enter the professional mental health community and are generally unmotivated for therapy. One of the positive features for these people is the nonprofessional atmosphere.

An important part of the success of "other-than-therapy" groups, particularly those that encourage members to become leaders, is the sharing with and caring for others. This form of "helper therapy" is described by Shaffer and Galinsky (1989). As group members make progress, they are encouraged to take on the role of helper or group leader. In the helper/leader role, feelings of dependence on others lessen and interpersonal competence increases.

By examining the principles developed by Shaffer and Galinsky to guide nonprofessional leaders, we can see how the role becomes therapeutic. The principles also demonstrate some of the ways the self-help group promotes change:

- Let members carry the group.
- Encourage older members to help newer members.
- Encourage all members to speak in every session.
- Remind group monopolizers that other members need a turn.
- Encourage members to speak from their heart rather than their head.
- Deter members from analyzing each others' hidden emotions.
- Encourage members to respond spontaneously.
- Model openness, spontaneity, empathy, and emotionality.
- Help members develop informal contracts for working on a problem behavior.
- Be willing to confront a problematic member.
- Develop times for socializing.
- Help the group develop norms and limits.

Note that intragroup differences and processes are not addressed; the emphasis is on survival skills, developing a social support network, and improving the present environment outside the group.

Whereas psychotherapy group leaders are very concerned about the group's compatibility and the patient/group match, support and self-help groups and 12-step groups have minimal admissions criteria and less stringent enforcement of norms. Most members are welcome as long as they are struggling with the identified problem/issue. At the same time, these groups do have clear norms. The most commonly known are the rules of the 12-step programs.

The 12-steps provide for the development of a new language and way of thinking. They are highly structured group norms that reflect the group's belief system. New members must be able and willing to follow the rules. The norms can attract or discourage members and become an important aspect of the group selection process. Unlike therapy groups, the 12 steps are not theoretically grounded but are pragmatic and often based on a spiritual perspective.

COMBINING PSYCHOTHERAPY AND "OTHER-THAN-THERAPY" GROUPS

"Other-than-psychotherapy" groups can be useful to psychotherapy group members during various stages of their treatment process:

1. In the pretherapy phase, for individuals who have low awareness of their problems and how they affect others
2. In the therapy phase (group or individual), as an adjunct and enhancement to therapy
3. In the maintenance phase, as support for maintaining gains

Pretherapy Phase

Participation in self-help, support, or 12-step groups can be part of an initial awakening to the depth of one's problems. The process of self-recognition and experience in a helping group atmosphere can prepare individuals for the more intensive work required in the psychotherapy group. Through a process of connection to others, in a supportive atmosphere, a way may be paved toward psychotherapy and the identification of broader therapeutic goals.

Psychotherapy

In later phases, self-help and 12-step programs can be integrated with psychotherapy to offer a patient broader support for therapeutic change. Matano and Yalom (1991) point out that traditional psychotherapy has failed alcoholics, many of whom have been helped by AA. The AA emphasis on sobriety as the primary goal has been neglected in psychotherapy. Many psychotherapeutic approaches have conceptualized chemical dependency in a nondisease model, which is incompatible with 12-step programs. Other conceptual differences as well have put the psychotherapies at odds with 12-step models. The spiritual emphasis of the approach and the 12 principles themselves seem to shift the responsibility for behavior away from the individual; while psychotherapy tends to focus directly on the individual's responsibility. However, Matano and Yalom provide a convincing model that integrates the interpersonal psychotherapy approach with AA's 12-steps approach.

Five principles can guide the clinician integrating the approaches and highlights how they can be combined.

1. The treatment priority must be recovery. This recognizes the main goals of AA. All the group's resources need to be mobilized toward abstinence, and the therapist must be very sensitive to threats to the recovery process. AA slogans such as "Don't analyze, utilize" seem to be antitherapeutic, but they are not, in fact. In the therapeutic context, the slogan suggests the need to avoid interpersonal analysis until the recovering alcoholic can tolerate—without recourse to alcohol—the anxiety that occurs when interpersonal behaviors are confronted.

2. The group members must identify as alcoholics. This encourages common goals among them and confronts their main resistance to therapy, their denial of the fact of their chemical dependency.

3. The group members' anxieties must be carefully regulated by the therapist. Alcoholics have used alcohol to cope with anxiety-evoking events. As a result, many activities that are a normal part of psychotherapy groups will raise anxiety in alcoholics, such as self-disclosure, giving and receiving feedback, and so on. One of the goals of AA is to provide a strong nondrinking social support system that *avoids* direct confrontation as part of the group process.

4. The group member is responsible for the addictive behaviors. He or she is accountable for taking the first drink, for relating to others in the present moment, and for the behaviors outlined in the 12 steps. These include self-understanding, making amends, carrying the AA message, and having faith.

5. Group psychotherapy techniques must be modified to integrate the values and beliefs of AA. AA meetings are highly structured and include specific roles, topics, and readings. Contributions are made to the group as a whole rather than to individual members. The structure is needed to help the alcoholic develop dependency on "people, places, or things." The nonprofessional leadership highlights the group bonding and creation of fellowship with those who have known the same struggle. Other recovering alcoholics provide a strong sense of hope and support for abstinence. Matano and Yalom suggest that the reliance on spirituality and prayer can be understood in a broader perspective to include reliance on others. In the psychotherapy group, the leader works with group members' loss-of-control difficulties often expressed as defiance, ego inflation, and counter dependency.

If the 12-step experience is not fully integrated with the psychotherapy group experience, a combined intervention can lead to problems. A group member may feel in conflict between 12-step and psychotherapy principles. Splitting may occur if the 12-step experiences and values are not discussed in the therapy group. Conversely, if the issue of responsibility is not explored, group members may avoid confronting their own behavior and how it affects others. The model described by Matano and Yalom indicates that when the two approaches are adequately combined, it is possible to treat the alcoholic successfully.

Maintenance Phase

Peer support groups and professionally led support groups can be useful as patients move into a maintenance phase. This is one of the most neglected areas of psychotherapy. How to maintain the changes attained in therapy is not systematically addressed in the psychotherapy literature. However, clinical evidence suggests that support groups are helpful to people who have made life-style changes, such as quitting a chemical dependency or eating disorder. Support groups for former patients, such as Anorexia Nervosa and Associated Disorders (ANAD) for eating-disordered patients, provide support for maintaining the changed behaviors and responding to relapses.

CONCLUSION

The clinician is influenced in selecting the appropriate group intervention for a patient by the fit between patient and group factors. The therapist takes into account where the patient is in the change process, the severity and nature of the patient's problem, and the patient's motivation for group therapy and tries to match them up with one among the wide range of group interventions, recognizing how each responds to patients' conceptualizations of their problems. The goal is not the perfect match, but the best possible match given the multiple patient and group factors that must be considered. The challenge is comparable to a search for Cinderella with more than one glass slipper.

REFERENCES

Alonso, A., & Swiller, H. I. (1993). Introduction: The case for group therapy. In A. Alonso & H. I. Swiller (Eds.), *Group therapy in clinical practice* (pp. xxi–xxv). Washington, DC: American Psychiatric Press.

Baker, M. N., & Baker, H. S. (1993). Self psychological contributions to the theory and practice of group psychotherapy. In A. Alonso & H. I. Swiller (Eds.), *Group therapy in clinical practice* (pp. 49–68). Washington, DC: American Psychiatric Press.

Beckett, A., & Rutan, J. S. (1990). Treating persons and AIDS in group psychotherapy. *International Journal of Group Psychotherapy, 40*, 19–29.

Brabender, V. M. (1985). Time-limited inpatient group therapy: A developmental model. *International Journal of Group Psychotherapy, 35*, 373–390.

Breier, A., & Strauss, J. S. (1984). The role of social relationships in the recovery from psychotic disorders. *American Journal of Psychiatry, 141*, 949–955.

Dies, R. R. (1993). Research on group psychotherapy: An overview and clinical applications. In A. Alonso & H. I. Swiller (Eds.), *Group therapy in clinical practice* (pp. 473–518). Washington, DC: American Psychiatric Press.

Drob, S., & Bernard, H. S. (1986). Time-limited group treatment of genital herpes patients. *International Journal of Group Psychotherapy, 36*, 133–144.

Flores, P. J. (1993). Group psychotherapy with alcoholics, substance abusers, and adult children of alcoholics. In H. I. Kaplan & B. J. Sadock (Eds.), *Comprehensive group psychotherapy* (3rd ed.). Baltimore, MD: Williams & Wilkins.

Gilligan, C., Rogers, A. G., & Tolman, D. L. (Eds.). (1990). *Women, girls, and psychotherapy: Reframing resistance.* Binghamton, NY: Harrington Park Press.

Herman, J., & Schatzow, E. (1984). Time-limited group therapy for women who have a history of incest. *International Journal of Group Psychotherapy, 34*, 605–616.

Huston, K. (1986). A critical assessment of the efficacy of women's groups. *Psychotherapy, Theory, Research and Training, 23*, 283–290.

Kanas, N. (1990). Short-term therapy groups for schizophrenics. In R. A. Wells & V. J. Giannetti (Eds.), *Handbook of the brief therapies* (pp. 551–564). New York: Plenum Press.

Kepner, J. I. (1987). *Body process: Working with the body in psychotherapy.* Cleveland: Gestalt Institute Press.

Kibel, H. D. (1992). The clinical application of object relations theory. In R. H. Klein, H. S. Bernard, & D. L. Singer (Eds.), *Handbook of contemporary group psychotherapy: Contributions from object relations, self-psychology, and social systems theories* (pp. 141–176). Madison, CT: International Universities Press.

Kibel, H. D. (1993). Inpatient group psychotherapy. In A. Alonso & H. I. Swiller (Eds.), *Group therapy in clinical practice* (pp. 93–111). Washington, DC: American Psychiatric Press.

Kipper, D. A. (1992). Psychodrama: Group psychotherapy through role playing. *International Journal of Group Psychotherapy, 42*, 495–521.

Kivlighan, D. M. (1985). Feedback in group psychotherapy: Review and implications. *Small Group Behavior, 16*, 373–385.

Klein, R. H. (1985). Some principles of short-term group psychotherapy. *International Journal of Group Psychotherapy, 35*, 309–330.

Knobloch, F., & Knobloch, J. (1979). *Integrated psychotherapy.* New York: Jason Aronson.

Krugman, S., & Osherson, S. (1993). Men in group therapy. In A. Alonso & H. I. Swiller (Eds.), *Group therapy in clinical practice* (pp. 393–420). Washington, DC: American Psychiatric Press.

Lazerson, J. S. (1984). Voices of bulimia: Experiences in integrated psychotherapy. *Psychotherapy: Theory, Research and Practice, 21*, 500–509.

Lazerson, J. S. (1986). Integrated psychotherapy at the Day house. *Psychiatric Annals, 16*, 709–714.

Lazerson, J. S., & Zilbach, J. J. (1993). Gender issues in group psychotherapy. In H. I. Kaplan & B. J. Sadock (Eds.), *Comprehensive group psychotherapy* (3rd ed., pp. 682–693). Baltimore, MD: Williams & Wilkins.

Leszcz, M., Yalom, I. D., & Norden, M. (1985). The value of inpatient group psychotherapy: Patients' perceptions. *International Journal of Group Psychotherapy, 35*, 411–433.

Lieberman, M. A. (1990). A group therapist perspective on self help groups. In M. Seligman & L. E. Marshak (Eds.), *Group psychotherapy: Interventions with special populations* (pp. 1–18). Needham Heights, MA: Allyn & Bacon.

Lieberman, M. A. (1993). Self-help groups. In H. I. Kaplan & B. J. Sadock (Eds.), *Comprehensive group psychotherapy* (3rd ed., pp. 292–304). Baltimore, MD: Williams & Wilkins.

Luborsky, L., Diguer, L., Luborsky, E., McLellan, A. T., Woody, G., & Alexander, L. (1993). Psychological health-sickness (PHS) as a predictor of outcomes in dynamic and other psychotherapies. *Journal of Consulting and Clinical Psychology, 61*, 542–548.

Mackenzie, K. R. (1987). Therapeutic factors in group psychotherapy: A contemporary view. *Group, 11*, 26–34.

Mackenzie, K. R. (1993). Time-limited group theory and technique. In A. Alonso & H. I. Swiller (Eds.), *Group therapy in clinical practice* (pp. 423–447). Washington, DC: American Psychiatric Press.

Matano, R. A., & Yalom, I. D. (1991). Approaches to chemical dependency: Chemical dependency and interactive group therapy—a synthesis. *International Journal of Group Psychotherapy, 41*, 269–293.

Piper, W. F., McCallum, M., & Azim, H. F. A. (1993). *Adaption to loss through short-term group psychotherapy*. New York: Guilford Press.

Oakley, A. (1992, February). *Womens' spaces: A framework for time-limited women's groups*. Paper presented at the American Group Psychotherapy Association Annual Conference, New York.

Rice, C. A., & Rutan, J. S. (1981). Boundary maintenance in inpatient therapy groups. *International Journal of Group Psychotherapy, 31*, 297–309.

Rutan, J. S., & Stone, W. N. (1993). *Psychodynamic group psychotherapy* (2nd ed.). New York: Guilford Press.

Salvendy, J. T. (1993). Selection and preparation of patients and organization of the group. In H. I. Kaplan & B. J. Sadock (Eds.), *Comprehensive group psychotherapy* (3rd ed., pp. 72–84). Baltimore, MD: Williams & Wilkins.

Scrignar, C. B. (1990). Group therapy with victims of post-traumatic stress disorder. In M. Seligman & L. E. Marshak (Eds.), *Group psychotherapy with special populations* (pp. 33–54). Needham Heights, MA: Allyn & Bacon.

Shaffer, J., & Galinsky, M. D. (1989). *Models of group therapy* (2nd ed.). Englewood Cliffs, NJ: Prentice Hall.

Vinogradov, S., & Yalom, I. D. (1989). *A concise guide to group psychotherapy.* Washington, DC: American Psychiatric Press.

Whiston, S. C., & Sexton, T. L. (1993). An overview of psychotherapy outcome research: Implications for practice. *Professional Psychology: Research and Practice, 24,* 43–51.

Yalom, I. D. (1983). *Inpatient group psychotherapy.* New York: Basic Books.

Yalom, I. D. (1985). *The theory and practice of group psychotherapy* (3rd ed.). New York: Basic Books.

SEVEN

USING THEORIES OF GROUP THERAPY

Elaine Cooper Lonergan

When I was supervising a student on his therapy group and introducing him to the theories of group therapy, he said, "You remind me of my violin teacher when I was a little boy. She would say, "Put the violin down; let's talk about music. What makes music?'" Now I was asking him, "What makes a group?"

We all know when we are part of a group but can we explain what that special ingredient is that makes it happen? Is it in the realm of art and mysticism and, therefore, impossible to explain? Would it help if we looked at the smallest group we can think of (Is the mother–child dyad a group?) and the largest (Is society a group?) and compare the two? Does a group become a group when each person surrenders a piece of themselves to the collective in order to obtain the gift of belonging? If so, what part of psychic structure do people share with the group: ego, id, superego, ego ideal, narcisissim? Does a group have to have a leader or a common purpose?

These are questions theorists have tried to answer. In this chapter I will look at their ideas, see how they fit with my own, and test their usefulness. Theories are relevant to group leaders in three ways: (1) they help organize data that otherwise would be overwhelming, (2) they generate new ideas for group interventions, (3) having a theory increases confidence that therapists know what they are doing; patients pick up on this and increase their engagement in the therapeutic process. Marmor (1988) found that therapists who were zealous about a theory and explained it to their patients got better results than those who did not. It did not matter what the theory was.

How do theorists answer the question, "What is a group?" Most believe a group has to have a leader to be a group. The leader may not be readily apparent, but he/she is there. Sometimes, the leader takes the form of a "common purpose."

Most theorists believe that each individual gives up a piece of their "I" to become a "we" but there is disagreement as to what part of the psychic structure is involved.

The mother–child dyad is not considered to be a group by everyone, but it is by Sigmund Freud (1921). He writes that a baby is born totally egocentric and it is only his group affiliation (his relationship with primary figures) that modifies his narcissism. His earliest group experiences civilizes him.

Society and religion are not considered to be groups by everyone, but they are by Eric Erikson (1980). He contends that these are major group affiliations that help to shape character. We learn through our culture which behavior will be valued by others. Since we need status from others to feed our self-esteem, and since basic self-esteem is a requirement for mental health, we are heavily influenced by the rewards our society grants.

If the definition of groups includes the relationship with mother as well as religious and national groups, then the list of groups in between must be endless. The more one thinks about it, the more groups one will think of (e.g., adolescent peer groups, sibling groups, work groups, etc.). The list goes on and on; just thinking about it can be overwhelming. This is where theory comes in. Theory helps organize these data and simplify them, so that the information can be grasped better. This does not mean theory equals the truth. A theory is simply an idea that gives *the feeling* of understanding (which is different from *actual* understanding).

Students interested in becoming group therapists often say, "There is too much to learn; too much goes on to comprehend; how can we track so many dynamics at one time—the group, eight individuals, the cotherapist, the setting? How do we know when to intervene?" Again, theory helps organize the process observed in the group, suggesting an idea about how to intervene. You can make the intervention and see what happens. If new material comes out in the group after the intervention, it can be considered positive. If the interaction becomes stultified, you can pull from another theory and make a different kind of intervention. This line of pursuit is modeled after Popper's (1968) scientific approach. He writes

> . . . there is the testing of the theory by way of empirical applications
> of the conclusions which can be derived from it. . . . The purpose of

this last kind of test is to find out how far the new consequences of the theory . . . stand up to the demands of practice. . . . With the help of other statements, previously accepted, certain singular statements—which we may call "predictions"—are deduced from the theory; especially predictions that are easily testable or applicable. Next we seek a decision as regards these (and other) derived statements by comparing them with the results of practical applications and experiments . . . if the singular conclusions turn out to be . . . verified, then the theory has, for the time being, passed its test. . . . (p. 33)

The game of science is, in principle, without end. He who decides one day that scientific statements do not call for any further test, and that they can be regarded as finally verified, retires from the game. (p. 53)

In this chapter, I will present seven theories that I have found useful in my work. I will share an example of group process from one of my own groups and analyze it through the lens of each theory. By asking the questions each theory tries to address, I will try to determine what novel interventions could be made.

Following are my process notes from a session of a therapy group of bulimic women. I will refer to this vignette throughout the chapter.

THE THERAPY SESSION

Mary recounts a dream in which she is leading the group in a parade through the city. Everyone is joyous. In the next fragment, she is alone with one of the therapists; the therapist is fondling her. She is toying with her and touching her in places that are not quite right. Mary is uncomfortable. Suddenly, Mary and the therapist hear Lilli, another group member, vomiting. Both the therapist and Mary run to help Lilli.

Some of the group members associate to the dream in the following ways: (1) Diane says that she felt competitive with Mary—she wanted to be the leader of the parade; (2) members express understanding of Mary's discomfort with the therapist, who sometimes "toys" with them and is insensitive; (3) Ann says that bulimia is sick behavior and it saved Mary from an uncomfortable situation; and (4) members see that disaster occurred when a member tried to take the leader's place.

Jane relates the dream to her relationship with her roommate. Jane was very angry with her roommate when she went out with Jane's boyfriend. The boyfriend then rejected Jane—but the roommate decided to put friendship with Jane first and rejected him. Lilli states factually that she guesses everyone has homosexual as well as heterosexual feelings and that the leader did not address the sexual part of the dream.

There is a pause. Members comment on Jane's change of appearance. She looks ravishing. She is wearing makeup for the first time and her face has a glow. She tells about the events of her week.

After the last meeting, Jane had her first homosexual encounter; it was with her roommate. The two of them went to a party where her ex-boyfriend was. They came home. They had been drinking. They hugged and kissed and lay in bed together. Before falling asleep the roommate told her that she was beautiful. Jane believed it because it was her roommate who said it. She felt wonderful. Her angry, competitive, jealous feelings toward her roommate disappeared and she continued to feel beautiful and wonderful until the group meeting.

Diane says she is jealous of Jane for having a homosexual encounter; she has always wanted to experiment. Lilli says she is glad to hear that others have had such wishes. They all say that they understand how a homosexual encounter can take bad, competitive feelings away, and they think that is terrific.

Kim, a new member, says she is worried about how the therapist feels about being attacked for "toying" with them. She knows that the therapist said she felt closer to Mary as a result of Mary's exposure of feelings, but Kim finds this hard to believe. Others say that they believed the therapist but feel the therapist has other feelings that she has not disclosed. For example, the therapist did not share her reaction to the sexual part of the dream. The therapist asks what their guesses are about her reaction. Some feel the therapist would be disgusted because she is obviously straight. Others think the therapist would be flattered. The therapist says, "That makes sense, since it is a compliment." The therapist continues, "It would be understandable for people here to have attractions for one another since sexuality is part of intimacy. And in this group everyone is attractive, intelligent, and interesting."

Jane says that she really looks forward to the group because the people are so neat. She adds that sometimes the therapist has the look of a sex kitten. Everyone laughs and says they know the look she is referring to.

Mary says that she feels attracted to Diane. Diane is shocked and squeals with glee. Lilli says that she also is attracted to Diane; she is perfectly proportioned and seems to be oblivious to her beauty. Diane is beside herself with joyful shock. She had been feeling like a "fat geek" all week. She went to a party and felt completely out of place. Others tell her that she must be doing something to push men away since she is so appealing.

Mary says that since she has stopped bingeing and vomiting, she has been overwhelmed with sexual desire. She never thought she could be the aggressor sexually but now she is constantly seducing her boyfriend.

Lilli says she thought she was frigid until she got her divorce and cut down her bingeing and vomiting; then she was ready to grab men off the street. Diane says she is closest with a gay, male friend and would like to sleep with him. Lilli says that she tried that and it did not work.

Cheryl says that she knows what Jane means—that aligning herself with her roommate made the competitive feelings go away. She had a similar experience with her best girlfriend. Mary says it is really funny, but since they have been talking about their homosexual attractions in the group, the competitive feelings she had in the dream have gone away. She is relieved. The therapist says that she makes it sound as though being competitive is a bad thing. They all say that it is. The therapist asks, "Why?" They say that one person wins, the others get stepped on. The therapist questions, "Why does *one* person have to win?" Members look puzzled. The therapist continues, "You make it sound as if there isn't room here for everyone at the top."

FREUD'S GROUP PSYCHOLOGY

In Freud's day, theorists such as LeBon (1920) and McDougall (1920) were making guesses as to why mobs (large groups) went out of control. Good people, when part of a mob, could act as animals. The theorists suggested that a "group mind" was created and it swallowed up people's judgment. In modern language, we could say that the members gave up their superego to the mob leader, letting the group leader set their moral standards. But why? Freud answered this question by going back to "Totem and Taboo" and "The Primal Horde."

We all have an unconscious memory of primal man; it is part of our collective unconscious. Here we find a father/chieftain who is self-centered and mean. He persecutes his sons with equal intensity. Freud (1921) speculated that the sons killed the father out of hatred and jealousy; a new leader emerged and the same murder took place. This pattern would eventually lead to the obliteration of the human race. Group formation was the solution. The group contained the murderous rage at and envy of the leader's women and riches. Following is a description of the primal horde and "kill the leader" behavior.

> [In] the scientific myth of the father of the primal horde . . . he was the ideal of each one of them, at once feared and honored. . . . These many individuals eventually banded together, killed him and cut him to pieces. None of the group of victors could take his place, or, if one of them did, the battles began afresh, until they understood that they must all renounce their father's heritage. They then formed the

totemic community of brothers, all with equal rights and united by
the totem prohibitions which were to preserve and expiate the
memory of the murder. (Freud, 1921, pp. 86–87)

How did the group contain these dangerous impulses? The wish to kill
the leader was replaced by making the hated leader the member's ego
ideal and identifying with him. Members identified with each other because they all had the same father/ego ideal. They assured themselves
that the leader, whose sole attention they wanted, would love or punish
them equally. With this understanding, they made a pact to stop killing
each other and their lust and aggression was contained.

Agazarian and Peters (1981) have suggested that there is a stage of
development in which maturing, complex groups go through a necessary phase of "killing the leader off." This stage is painful for members
and leaders since the most primitive urges are stimulated and relived.
Only strong groups and people can endure the torment and move on to
the next stage of maturity. Here is their description of the phase:

> Primal horde dynamics . . . wish to consume the leader in order to
> incorporate his power. . . . Oral and sadistic fantasies are aroused;
> annihilation and pre-oedipal castration anxiety is experienced. (p. 138)

They describe a student's emotional reaction when experiencing this
phase with his group:

> To his surprise he had experienced the kind of terror that would have
> been appropriate had he really been about to be killed or eaten.
> (p. 138)

Unlike LeBon, McDougall and Freud did not agree that all people
regressed in all groups (Rutan & Stone, 1993). Freud felt that groups
could also be positive in that people could temporarily give up their
neuroses. The level of the regression in the group could be controlled
by (1) increasing structure in the group, (2) decreasing the size of the
group, and (3) members' identification with the leader (Scheidlinger,
1980). These have all been useful ideas in developing a knowledge base
for the practice of group therapy.

As noted earlier, Freud also acknowledged the importance of group
affiliation from the beginning of personality development. He saw no
difference between individual and group psychology. The separation
between them has been devised for our convenience, so that we will not
be too confused by complexity.

Before we apply Freud's theory to group process and create possible interventions, let me remind you that Freud saw the group as civilizing the impulse-ridden (sexual and aggressive), egocentric individual.

Analysis

Now I will go back to the group process notes that I presented in the introduction. In order to look at the material through the lens of this theory, I need to ask the following questions: Can I find contained aggression and "kill the leader or sibling instinct?" Do I get a glimpse of the rivalry and murderous rage that is beneath the manifest content of the group? Do I want to make an intervention that will help the members achieve conscious awareness of their rage? Is the leader functioning as an ego ideal? What is the size and structure of the group? Do I want to alter either to get more or less regression in the group?

My analysis of the vignette from the perspective of Freudian theory is: Bulimics are usually bulimic to hide primitive feelings because they are so frightened of them. Part of the therapy group leader's task is to help members be less frightened of rage and sexuality so that they can give up bulimia as a defense. In this group session, the killer instinct and sexual drive of the members is fairly close to the surface, possibly because the leader has encouraged expression of such feeling and created a safe environment to explore them. One can see how such feelings are coming to the surface (Mary dethrones the leader and takes her place in the group and others admit that they would like to do the same; they all admit to homosexual longings including seeing the therapist as a sex object) and their fear of such feelings (Mary uses bulimia to stop her wish to take over the group; certain members use sexual attraction to halt their hatred of the other; Kim is frightened of the effect of expressed anger toward the therapist). At the end of the session, members are explicit about their fear that one member will win the competition and the others will be killed off. The leader understands this fear but tries to replace it with another construct: Maybe they can all win. In other words, now that the group is aware of their primal horde memory and how it affects their perceptions, they can begin to test the reality of this fearful expectation.

The leader is a strong ego ideal for all the members, which leads to group formation. What she says is important to everyone. The leader is satisfied with the degree of regression in the group, she thinks it is just what they can handle.

If Freud's group psychology were applied to this group more rigorously, the leader could be explicit about the unconscious material that is emerging. When members finish their associations to Mary's dream, the leader could say: "The wish to kill me off and to step on each other in order to take my place is so frightening that it feels safer to be bulimic and get such a thought out of mind."

When Jane describes her sexual encounter with her roommate and how wonderful it was, the leader could say, "It seems as though being sexual for the first time with a woman was less frightening to you than thoughts of wanting to murder your roommate for betraying you." And when the members are enjoying their sexual attraction to one another, the leader could say, "I can see you are all enjoying your sexuality right now, and I wonder if you could accept your murderous impulses at the same time."

BASIC ASSUMPTION THEORY

It is not uncommon to be sitting in a staff meeting and finding it almost impossible to stay focussed on the task at hand. The purpose of the meeting may be to figure out how to see more people in the same amount of time, but the staff group is arguing about whether to have a coffee machine. The leader of the group must constantly redirect the members in order to get anything accomplished. Why do work/task groups have so much trouble staying focussed? Wilfred Bion tried to answer this question.

Bion postulated that people in a group are always torn between working on the task at hand and an unconscious basic assumption about why the group is together. Members have a conscious purpose for attending a meeting, but their collective unconscious has a different agenda. Unconscious agenda are aimed at gratifying primitive desires. Members collude in an unconscious, out-of-awareness process in which the group acts *as if* it is meeting for a different purpose (Rioch, 1970).

Bion postulated three basic assumptions: dependency, fight/flight, and pairing. In the *dependency basic assumption*, group members act as if they are helpless, dumb, and immature and the leader is omniscient. If the members are patient, the leader will come forth with some magic and save them. The group might offer up a sick member in order to test the leader. The members do not really care about the suffering member; they are using the person to get what they need from the leader. The members' expectations of the leader are so high that the leader has to fail. The frustration in the group keeps building.

In the *flight/fight basic assumption*, the group meets to fight or flee from an enemy. The leader is needed to find the enemy and then lead the group into or away from battle. The individual members do not matter to anyone; if a few get trampled on in the fighting or fleeing, it is acceptable. There is no room for sick or weak members. Members are anti-intellectual and anti-introspective. They have no frustration toler-ance. What matters is the preservation of the group and the need *to act.*

Hope is the hallmark of the *pairing basic assumption.* In this assump-tion, the group is waiting for a messiah to save it. It is important that the messiah never actually come; members *are waiting* for redemption. The group becomes interested in some couple in the group and joke about their sexuality, because the assumption is that this couple will give birth to the messiah. The messiah might come in the form of a new idea or some other form of creation.

These basic assumptions may sound familiar to you. They actually parallel oral, anal, and oedipal primary process. They also represent parts of the unconscious that people often want to disavow, which explains why they remain unconscious.

A basic assumption operates in all groups, and in some instances it helps with task completion. For example: The dependency basic assump-tion helps the church, which is based on worshipping and depending upon a higher being; the fight/flight basic assumption helps the army, which is organized around fighting an enemy; the pairing basic assump-tion helps the aristocracy because subjects will become emotionally involved in the king and queen and the progeny they produce (note the investment people have in the activities of Prince Charles and Princess Diana and how this investment could help them rule).

Bion conjectures that although we have a capacity for all the basic assumptions each of us has our own "valency" (tendency or affinity) toward one or another. The basic assumption of a group is the one held by the majority of members.

Analysis

Now I will go back to my process notes and consider what basic assump-tion the group is operating from. Can I assess the valency of the group members? Would it help the group for me to make the unconscious con-scious by interpreting their process? Does the group's basic assumption help further the task at hand?

My analysis of this vignette from a Bionian perspective is that this group seems to be, or is trying to be, in the pairing basic assumption, based on the tone of sexual excitement and optimism in the session (rep-resented by Jane coming to the group looking ravishing). The group fantasizes that if the leader would pair with a group member (as presented in the dream when the leader and Mary are physically intimate), greater freedom would be produced for the group members. This freedom includes the opportunity to have a satisfying sexual relationship. The leader represents mental health and the group member represents the bulimic pathology; when these two wed, the strengths and weaknesses of each member can become integrated.

The pairing basic assumption actually helps the group therapist with her task. She wants the members to fantasize about genital sexuality because this is an area that causes trepidation for them. In fact, much of the eating disorder pathology stems from fear of sexual development.

The therapist also wants the group to be hopeful about their condition. Yalom (1995) considers hope one of the curative factors; it is especially important for these women whose bulimia is often fueled by depression. So the leader makes interventions that encourage the women to develop a pairing basic assumption. For example, she conveys that she is flattered by members seeing her as a sexual being and that she is not put off by the idea of sexual play with a group member. At the end of the meeting, she hints that the members have good reason to be optimistic; after all, they can all compete for sexual partners and they can all win their prize.

Further interventions the group leader could make if she were using Bion's basic assumption theory would be to say explicitly: "If Mary and I have a private liaison, maybe we could produce a baby that was mentally healthy but also had the sensitivity one achieves through knowing the suffering of bulimia." Or later in the meeting, when optimism and play were flourishing with Jane's glow and mutual admiration, the leader might say, "Yes, rebirth is in the air. New selves are being born here."

GROUP FOCAL CONFLICT THEORY

Whitaker and Lieberman (1964) systematically studied tapes of group meetings, looking at the manner in which conversation developed. One person would speak and then another, but what did the second member pick up on from the first? And the third from the second? A pattern seemed to develop from one speaker to the next. But how did the group create the pattern or choose what the topic of the day would be? The researchers concluded that group members joined to solve one unconscious conflict after another in order to alleviate tension and anxiety, and they called the conflict the *group focal conflict*. This conflict always contains a wish (the *disturbing motive*) and a fear (the *reactive motive*). The group's solution is either *enabling*—part of the wish (and its accompanying anxiety) can be realized—or *restrictive*—no part of the wish is allowed gratification (and thus no anxiety is experienced). Once the group finds a solution, members go on to a new conflict. The theme of the group consists of a series of focal conflicts united by the same *disturbing motive* (wish). The culture of the group arises from the pattern in which the group solves conflicts (Whitman & Stock, 1980).

The technique suggested by Whitaker and Lieberman involves the group therapist leading the group toward enabling solutions. The therapist composes a group of members whose capacities for anxiety tolerance are similar; the therapist assesses how much anxiety the group members can tolerate; the therapist then suggests solutions with the optimal degree of anxiety that the members can tolerate. The therapist can talk to the group through an intervention with an individual member or the therapist can talk to the individual member through a group-as-a-whole intervention. It is important that the therapist do everything possible to establish and maintain a safe environment so that members do not feel judged; in this way, members can take risks in discovering enabling solutions.

Analysis

Now I must go back to my process notes and ask the following questions: What is the group wish? The group fear? What kind of solution does the group use—enabling or restrictive? Does the leader suggest a solution or help the group move toward an enabling or restrictive solution? Does the leader talk to the group through the individual intervention or an individual through group intervention? Is the group composed of people who can tolerate the same degree of anxiety? Is the environment of the group safe and nonjudgmental? What interventions could I make if I followed this model?

My analysis of the vignette from the perspective of focal conflict theory is that Mary's dream presents two focal conflicts for the group: the wish to have an exclusive sexual alliance with the group leader and the wish to replace her as the leader of the group. The fear is that the other group members would kill her if either wish were realized. The solution in the dream is that sickness keeps Mary from her wishes; gratification of the wishes ceases to be possible as soon as bulimic behavior begins. In the group, however, members do allow themselves some gratification of the wishes: They are able to talk about their difficult feelings. Diane acknowledges a similar wish to Mary's—a desire to lead the group— and the group sees that they ordinarily would choose to get sick rather than face their fear of competition. Members then try another solution: if they join together in a sexual alliance, like Jane and her roommate, they will not kill each other and they can gratify some of their sexual impulses. Kim expresses the fear: Perhaps the leader will not approve of their sexuality. Here the leader encourages the enabling solution by suggesting that she is not threatened by their sexual fantasies of her; in fact, she is flattered by them. The group responds to this intervention by enjoying homosexual play. Members then take the risk of admitting to heterosexual desires. They stay on this subject briefly because of their fear of competing with each other. The group members are clear about their wish and the leader helps them to clarify their fear. The fear is agreed on: Only one person can win the race; everyone else loses (they are killed off). The fear is catastrophic because they all need the affectional bonds they have formed. The leader questions the reality basis of their fear and opens up new possibilities for them.

One senses in this group a high level of safety. Wishes and fears emerge easily; members trust each other. Members also trust the therapist and use her help to find more enabling solutions. The group seems to be composed of members who have similar degrees of anxiety tolerance; all of the members participate in the discussion. No one runs out of the room or disassociates.

The leader could have made more explicit interventions during the session. After Mary presented her dream, the therapist could have said: "Probably each of you has the desire to have the therapist to yourself and to lead the group, but you have stopped such thoughts because the consequences would be severe." Or, later in the session, when the group noted how their competitive feelings dissipated with sexuality, she could have said to the whole group: "What is so bad about being competitive? What is so great about having such feelings go away?" On the other hand, she could have focused on Jane and worked with her, knowing that her issue is also that of the group's. At the beginning of the meeting she could have focused on Mary, knowing that the dream reflects conflicts everyone in the group is experiencing.

LIVING SYSTEMS THEORY

A group is a living system, as is the cell of the body, the human organism, and society as a whole. Living systems theory, fathered by von Bertalanffy (1966), is a way of talking about all living systems in one set of terms. Instead of different vocabularies for biology, anthropology, psychiatry, and sociology, this theory attempts to develop a single, inclusive terminology. Systems theory is also a way of organizing the complex whole. Looking at the therapy group as a system, it clearly contains many systems, including suprasystems and subsystems (Durkin, 1975). For example, there is the system within which the group takes place—the agency, the cultural and societal systems that the agency functions in, the therapist system that organizes the group, each individual member system that participates, the psychic system that organizes each member, and the group-as-a-whole system. One can continue this list indefinitely. Few theories try to make sense out of this complex whirl; systems theory does.

Living systems share certain properties; the group as a whole has the same qualities as other living systems. System theorists argue that it is important for group therapists to analyze the health of their group's system and to learn how to doctor it when necessary.

Living systems are defined units, with boundaries, that are in continuous interaction within and without. They are constantly changing, yet maintain constancy; they are in "flux equilibrium" (fleiss gleichgewicht). They all have subsystems to execute certain functions and are part of a suprasystem. (In a therapy group the therapist is at the apex of the group system and serves as an organizing function.) The system is open and matures toward greater organization (negentropy) but it has limitations (equifinality). If a system is unhealthy, it will move toward randomness (entropy).

There is an *isomorphic connection between all the subsystems and the suprasystem*. With the therapy group, there is a resonance of themes and parallel process between each member system, the group system, the supervisor system, the agency system, the societal system, the therapist system, and so on. One can imagine how difficult it would be to try to figure out the isomorphic connections between and among these systems, but at least four authors have tried. Agazarian and Peters (1981) analyzed the isomorphic connections between the member, group-as-a-whole, person, and group-role systems. They looked at each system according to theory, communication behavior, norms, goals, roles, cohesiveness, and structure. Ashbach and Schermer (1987) mapped out the isomorphic connections between the intrapsychic system, the interactive system, and the group-qua-group system on the dimensions of (1) comprehensive views of object relations and the self; (2) affects/defenses; (3) identification and externalization; (4) phantasy; (5) cognitive mastery; (6) boundary and structure.

Certainly systems theory gives us a tool for approaching the complexity of the therapy group. It can deter us from taking too simplistic a view of the group process. It also explains the parallel process (the isomorphic connection) that is often mysterious but so useful to understand. One example is how supervisees can re-create in supervision what goes on in the group without being aware of it (students coming late to supervision and the supervisor feeling worthless vis-à-vis the same behavior in patients and group leaders). Another is how cotherapists can re-create in their private dialogue the conflict in the group without being aware of it (cotherapists who find themselves fighting over a petty issue realize that the group members have projected onto them their inadequacy, resulting in the group leaders starting to devalue each other). Another example is how intrapsychic conflicts can shape the group-as-a-whole process (anorexic patients create a value system in the group in which status is assigned by thinness.)

Systems theory helps us look at boundary functioning and ask whether systems' boundaries are too open or too closed. If they are too open, how do we help close them? If they are too closed, how do we help open them?

A group member whose boundary is too open can be one who merges with others, such as the codependent wife who focuses more on her husband's ups and downs than on her own. The therapist might help her look at her own emotional conflicts separate from her husband's by pushing for "I" statements. When the therapist facilitates the individuation process, it helps with boundary closing. A group member whose boundary is too closed can be one who is very obsessive. He ruminates on the same issues over and over again. The therapist might help him open his boundary by asking him to listen and repeat what another group member has said or to recount what is different in the group meeting room. Any new sensual, physical, or verbal experience helps new information get through the boundary; often just coming to the group (a new, impinging external system) loosens an individual's boundary.

An example of a therapy group that is too open is one in which people never come on time and members talk continuously about people outside the group. There is no sense of cohesion. The leader may help to close the boundary by ruling that people come each week and on time or they cannot be part of the group. The leader might insist that part of the group time be spent on here-and-now process—people talking about their feelings about each other in the moment. An example of a therapy group that is too closed is one that is so homogeneous that the process is repetitive and boring. Everyone agrees on everything, so there is no anxiety or tension in the group. The leader might help to open the system by bringing in new members or choosing to be withdrawn or confrontive, which will stress the group members. The leader could also shock the system. Minuchin (1978) and other family therapists who work with enmeshed families (very tight systems) write about various techniques to "shake up the system." For example, I once had a group of anorexics who created a tight, unhealthy system where they believed the perfect womb had been created in the group, and it was reasonable to expect total acceptance everywhere. I told one member that I did not care if she was frustrated when I took a vacation; in fact, I was glad. What the members heard was that I did not care, and the bubble in the group burst. It took them a year to understand that optimum frustration was a good thing for growth.

Analysis

Now I will refer to my example of group process and assess the health of the various systems, especially the boundary functioning. Can I see the various subsystems and the function they serve and the supersystems? Can I envision various boundary opening and closing techniques? Am I aware of the structure of the group—the norms, status system, culture? What about parallel process between the various systems? Can I define some of the isormorphic connections? My analysis of this vignette from a systems' theory perspective is that group therapy can work to alter individual systems. The person who is intact as a system comes into the group, which is a new system, opens up boundaries to let new information in, and is changed as a result.

The session starts with Mary's dream. The fact that it is about the group demonstrates that she has opened up the boundaries of her psychic system to the group system. In the sexual dream fragment, the boundary between therapist and patient breaks down too much and the patient experiences discomfort. The psyche protects itself by stopping this interaction and focusing on a sick member of the group. This protection mechanism resonates (the isomorphic connection) with other members' psyches and the group process since "focusing on others" and "people pleasing" is a central dynamic. With bulimics, this dynamic often goes to an extreme in which boundaries are too open and external system needs matter more than internal ones.

By going out with Jane's boyfriend, Jane's roommate did not respect boundaries. Jane was frightened by her hostility toward her roommate and used eroticism to soften it. In this way she could maintain communication (flow of information between two systems). At the same time, the entire group followed suit by using sexuality to make it safer to be open with each other and to suppress mutual hostility.

The remainder of the analysis focuses on the interaction between the member system of the group and the therapist system. The members reveal their discomfort with genuine homosexual and heterosexual feelings but test the leader to see if she agrees (they open up their boundaries to the leader's boundaries). The leader conveys approval and even delight with such basic drives, and the members start to incorporate her attitude. She also makes it safer for them by assuring them that no one will die in the process (they can all win). The leader, at the same time, is being influenced by the group and, in turn, her own system is changing. Perhaps she is not used to talking about homosexual feelings and is surprised at her pleasure in receiving sexual attention from the group members.

The members and group seem to be maintaining optimum boundary openness. The members are in anxiety-ridden waters but are able to handle it, as is the leader. The group is cohesive, and new intrapsychic and interpersonal material can be let in.

Further interventions that a systems therapist might make follow. (1) After Mary presents her dream, the therapist could say, "It is helpful when people bring in dreams about the group." This comment encourages other members to open the group and psyche systems for cross-fertilization. (2) When Jane presents her sexual encounter with her roommate after she had been betrayed, the leader could say, "I think, Jane, that you are struggling with some of the same issues in the group as you were with your roommate." The leader would be pointing out the isomorphic connection between Jane's inside-the-group and outside-the-group social systems. The leader could also suggest that Jane was "acting out"—letting spill over the group boundary a solution to a group problem. The leader could help the group close its boundaries and deal with interpersonal issues in the group, not elsewhere. (3) If members started to be physical with each other (e.g., seeing what it was like to kiss each other), the therapist might add structure or close boundaries. She might say, "This is group therapy and it is important that we use words rather than actions to describe our feelings."

FOULKES'S PSYCHOANALYSIS IN GROUPS

Foulkes (1948, 1975), a follower of Freud, was one of the first psychoanalysts to believe that it was possible to do psychoanalysis in groups. The primary tenets of psychoanalysis—the understanding and use of transference (where the patient experiences the analyst as a significant figure from the past) and resistance (to gaining insight and changing one's personality structure)—could be applied to groups, and the primary technique used in psychoanalysis—interpretation (making the unconscious conscious)—would lead to personal insight in members of groups as well as individuals. Foulkes believed in man's social nature and that all mental illness was due to problems in interpersonal relationships; for this reason relationships in a group setting could clarify intrapsychic conflict. In the group, members have transferences to other group members as well as to the group leader. Resistance occurs as members use a variety of ego defenses to protect against anxiety. The group members often operate as a whole (a group) and the group as a whole develops its own defenses against treatment.

Foulkes believed in the power of the group to be curative and felt that his role as therapist was simply to create the setting conducive to group formation. He "conducted" the group in the direction of birth and maturation, giving the group ample time to find its own way, and intervened only when he felt the group was going off the track of growth.

Influenced by Melanie Klein and object relations theory, Foulkes posited four levels of group process: (1) *Current level*: What is the reality level of the group—the setting of the group, the identity of leader and members, the circumstances of the group meeting? (2) *Transference level*: What are the transferences displayed by the group members? Member-to-member transferences? Member-to-therapist transferences? Group-as-a-whole transferences (how a member sees the group as a unit—as a mother? or father?)? (3) *Projective level*: What are the primitive part-objects that members project on one another? Is one member's anger seen in another and not in himself? Or his sexuality? Or love? Is someone being scapegoated: all the members projecting their despicable parts onto one person? and (4) *Primordial level*: What about the collective unconscious of the group? What are the archetypical shared images that no one talks about? The memory of totem and taboo? Feminine and masculine images?

Analysis

Now I will refer to my process notes. Where is transference taking place? Where is resistance operative? Where are the four levels of group process? How active is the group leader? Does the leader give the group a chance to solve a problem before he intervenes? Would the group or members benefit by the leader making the unconscious conscious?

My analysis of the vignette from the perspective of Foulkes is that each part of Mary's dream can be looked at as a separate part of Mary, and each character in the dream can therefore be seen as a projection. The therapist who toys with her can be construed as a projection of the part of her that manipulates people, while Lilli represents the sick part of her. The toying therapist could also be a transference object and represent her mother. It is only through Mary's associations that we can figure this out, and the leader does not explore this area.

Later, when Lilli states factually that everyone has homosexual and heterosexual feelings, she is acknowledging reality, but it also may link to a memory of humankind's struggle to be sexual but not kill for sex. This collective unconscious memory may also be connected to the members' fear of competition and the concomitant "killing each other off" (only one person can win the competition). Members seem to be struggling with integrating nondestructive sexuality into their self-image and their relationships. In this challenge they join hands with every human being on earth since the beginning of time.

Members refer to reality throughout the process when they report what has happened outside the group (Jane had her first homosexual encounter, Mary had a dream, Lilli feels more sexual). The reality or societal level of this group also includes the setting of the group—it is a private therapy group in San Francisco, the members work and pay for their treatment, members do not meet outside the group. This reality has relevance in understanding the group. The transference to the therapist may be more intense than in a clinic setting where it is shared with an institutional transference.

Continuing through the session, the therapist does not answer the members immediately when one of them asks her how she responded to the sexual part of the dream. Instead, she asks members for their associations, a tactic that is likely to bring unconscious material to the fore. Some members feel that the therapist will be disgusted by homosexual feelings, which could be attributed to projection (the members would be disgusted), transference (the members had parents who clearly were disgusted by sex), or both. Jane says that the therapist has the look of a sex kitten. This could be reality, transference (Jane having had a sexy parent), projection (she is feeling like a sex kitten—remember, she looks ravishing today), or some combination of these factors. The group seems to share the reaction formation defense against anxiety over competition (they love each other and therefore do not need to be angry and compete with each other).

The therapist is nondirective in this session, as Foulkes might recommend. There is plenty of space for the members to interact before the leader intervenes. When she does intervene, it is to move the process along. The members respond, indicating that a safe therapy environment has been provided.

Further interventions that a psychoanalytically trained group therapist might make are as follows. (1) After Mary presents her dream, the therapist could say, "I can see everyone can identify with Mary wanting to lead the group and Lilli bingeing and vomiting, but what about the therapist toying with Mary in an inappropriate manner? Is anyone in touch with that part of themselves?" The therapist would be helping members get in touch with the projective level of the group process. (2) When members are associating with how the therapist felt about being a sexual object, one member said she would be disgusted. The therapist could explore the possibility of a transference reaction by asking the members, "Who was the first person you can remember who was disgusted by sex?" (3) When Diane says that she was sure she was a "fat geek" all week and the group confirms that nothing could be further from the truth, the therapist could explore this contradiction. "It appears that you are seeing yourself as the opposite of how you are perceived. What gain could there be for you in seeing yourself as unattractive?" The therapist would be starting an attack on her defenses.

YALOM'S HERE-AND-NOW APPROACH

Yalom's popular textbook on group therapy (1985) has profoundly influenced group therapy practice in this country. Influenced by Harry Stack Sullivan (1953), who believed that pathology derives from interpersonal perceptual distortions, Yalom promulgates the here-and-now approach and believes that the therapist should facilitate interaction in the group. After the interaction develops, members are encouraged to look at their part in the interaction. Yalom calls this the "self-reflective loop": Interact and then look at it and learn from it. Members are discouraged from talking about their past or activities outside the group; what is important is that they look at their interaction in the here and now. Common interventions are "But what about right now in the group?" "How are you feeling about me right now?" These are usually hard questions to answer.

Since the group is a microcosm of society and the family, members act out their conflictual relationships in the present. This interaction is open to inspection by other group members and the leader. The members get feedback and are encouraged to try new behaviors.

Prior to writing the first edition of his text, Yalom looked at the literature and his own group experience and developed a list of "curative factors" in group therapy, the essential things that make people get better. He now calls them "therapeutic factors," and they are as follows:

• Instillation of hope
• Universality ("I am not alone")
• Imparting of information
• Altruism ("I can help others")
• Corrective recapitulation of the primary family group
• Development of socializing techniques
• Imitative behavior
• Interpersonal learning
• Group cohesiveness
• Catharsis
• Existential factors ("There are certain things such as loneliness and death that every human being has to face")

Note that group cohesiveness is one of the therapeutic factors. Yalom tries hard in his book to direct therapists in a manner that is most likely to produce a cohesive group: good preparation of members, optimal group composition, healthy group boundaries and norms, and so on. It is cohesiveness that causes members to cathect the group and take seriously what happens in it. It adds the magic to group therapy and to any "real" group experience. It is hard to describe it but everyone who has been a part of one knows what a cohesive group is. The group really matters to the members. The whole (group) is greater than the sum of its parts (the individual members).

Analysis

Now I will look at my group process notes and ask myself the following questions: Is the group cohesive? What are the curative factors operating in the group? Are the members or is the leader working in the here-and-now? Can I think of new interventions by applying the here-and-now approach?

My analysis of this vignette, based on Yalom's approach is that this group is cohesive, and its cohesiveness is demonstrated by the openness of the members. They are revealing material that they have told no one else. They have made the group a new family and are thus very influenced by the comments of other members and the group leader. This is a healthier family than they have known; they are participating in a corrective emotional experience. Members have found a haven in the group since they are all bulimic, and they have decided that they are all all right. They are not alone. They can give to each other. They are valued. They have learned that underlying their bulimic behavior are conflicts that most women struggle with: how to be beautiful and good so that those of importance will accept you; how to express anger, sadness, and fear without alienating the people you need and love.

Members are courageous in dealing with here-and-now feelings when they tell each other that they are sexually attracted to each other, that they are envious of another member leading the group or having a homosexual encounter, that they feel uncomfortable with some of the leader's interventions (she toys with them), and that they think the group leader looks sexy. It is not unusual for a flood of affect to emerge when someone says something in the here-and-now. In the group, the members respond enthusiastically when Jane says the leader looks like a sex kitten. Because members are exposing unconscious and conscious reactions to others in the group, they can test them out, get feedback and then modify them. Once the unconscious emerges, the ego, with the help of the group, can start to process and master it.

Note that the group spontaneously relates in the here-and-now, or at least it seems to. Even though the leader does not give any prompting, she has obviously educated this group in working effectively; she influenced the norms of the group in its formative stage.

Other here-and-now interventions the leader could have made are as follows: (1) When Jane describes the encounter with her roommate, the leader could ask, "What gut feelings are you people having as you listen to Jane? Just pick one word. Remember, feelings are anger, sadness, joy, fear, frustration, etc." (2)When Kim says that she is nervous about the therapist's reaction to sexual questions and others deny such a concern, the leader might say, "Wait a minute, don't dismiss this so quickly. If anyone shared Kim's concern, would you feel comfortable saying so?" (3) After Mary reports her dream, the leader could ask, "How was it for people to listen to a dream in here?" or "Have your feelings toward Mary changed since she brought in this dream?" or "Mary, how do you feel now—in the group—after sharing your dream?"

THE COGNITIVE/BEHAVIORAL APPROACH

Cognitive and behavioral approaches are combined in this chapter because neither are psychodynamic (concerned with the "why" of behaviors). Cognitive therapists are interested in the spontaneous thought processes of their patients. Behavior therapists try to change maladaptive behaviors. Both make the assumption that if certain negative thinking changes or if maladaptive behaviors change, the person will also change; that is, if you change one part of the system, the entire system will necessarily change.

Beck et al. (1979) discuss the rationale for cognitive therapy. They propose that one's affect and behavior are largely determined by cognitions; thought processes derive from attitudes and assumptions about former events and may not be appropriate to current circumstance. Ellis (1992) believes that people overgeneralize from childhood and often turn parental teaching into "shoulds," "oughts," and "musts." He gives examples of absolute must cognitions:

(1) "*I* (ego) *absolutely must* perform important tasks well and be approved by significant others or else I am an inadequate, worthless person!" (2) "*You* (other people) *must* treat me considerately and kindly or else you are a rotten person!" (3) "*Conditions* (my environment) *must* give me what I need and never greatly deprive me or else the world is a terrible place!" (p. 64)

An example of absolute should thinking is:

"Because I'm not performing as well as I *absolutely should*, it's *awful*, *I can't stand it*, I'm an *inadequate person*, and I'll *always* fail and *never* be competent and loveable." (p. 65)

Wolpe (1982), a pioneer of behavior therapy, writes that bad habits are learned; by studying the learning process, one can unlearn them. Reinforcement (rewards) is the way responses are acquired and existing ones threatened. Unlearning takes place when behavior stops being reinforced and eventually becomes extinct. It is important to identify the circumstances in which a behavior was originally conditioned (often in childhood), and the later events that modified it or led to its spread through second-order conditioning.

Therapy for groups that are composed of patients who have behavioral disturbances (e.g., as alcoholics, bulimics, substance abusers) should include behavioral and cognitive monitoring (Lonergan, 1984). In a group for bulimics, time should be spent finding out the frequency of bulimic episodes among the group members and whether the frequency is increasing or decreasing. Members should spend time sharing coping mechanisms and the details of how they have managed to curtail binges. Any decrease of the pathological behavior should be applauded.

Cognitive therapists ask patients to monitor the thoughts they have during the day and prior to certain activities. If a woman fails a test, how does she talk to herself? Does she say to herself: "What a dummy you are. You should have studied harder. You need to be punished for being bad. You can't spend any money today." Or does she say: "You may have failed but you did the best you could. You studied harder for this test than you have for any other. Though you didn't pass, you got closer to passing than you ever have. Even so, it is hard to fail; let's see what we can do to comfort you. How about a bubble bath tonight?"

Most people who are self-destructive have thought processes that are negative and self-recriminating; the depressed person will say that a glass with some water in it is half empty rather than half full. Furthermore, if you follow the person's thoughts during the day, you will find that the person sees everything in the most negative light.

Cognitive therapists try to change destructive thinking. They have developed such techniques as internal alarm setting. When one has a negative thought an alarm goes off that says, "STOP!" Then the person purposefully substitutes a healthier thought. He may have notes posted all over his house, in his office, in his car, reminding him of positive thoughts to think. The 12-step programs utilize such tools. Each morning members read positive aphorisms and try to remember them all day: "I am okay," "I wasn't born bad," "It is my parent's criticism I am hearing in my head, not my own."

Another cognitive tool is "relabeling," in which one reframes a perception. For example, a young woman feels guilty about not calling her mother every day. The voice in her head says, "You are a bad person for not calling your mother. It means that you do not love her, and you are ungrateful for all she has done for you." The same action can be reframed and relabeled: "Good, you haven't called your mother today. You are one step further along to being an independent, effective adult of whom you and your mother can be proud."

Beck et al. (1979) write that it is important to teach the patient (1) to monitor negative, automatic thoughts; (2) to recognize connections between cognition, affect, and behavior; (3) to examine evidence for and against distorted automatic thought; (4) to substitute more reality-oriented interpretation for biased cognitions; and (5) to learn to identify and alter dysfunctional beliefs that predispose the patient to distort experiences (p. 4). Homework assignments include the patient keeping a daily record of dysfunctional thoughts, an hourly activity report, a rating of each activity according to mastery and pleasure, and a list of tasks leading to a particular goal. Patients strive to look at their conclusions scientifically: What is the logic that led to the conclusion? The evidence is examined and alternatives considered. Experiments are designed to test the premises. For instance, if a patient believes that people turn away from him or her with disgust, a system for judging people's reactions is determined and recorded. Other techniques are cognitive rehearsal (where every step of the thinking process is reviewed and roadblocks identified), assertiveness training, and role playing.

Techniques that Wolpe (1982), a pioneer in behavior therapy, advocates include behavior rehearsal, operant conditioning, and systematic desensitization. In behavior rehearsal, patients act out scenes in their life and experiment with new forms of behavior. Systematic desensitization involves (1) induction of a calm state through muscle relaxation, (2) exposure to a weak version of the avoided stimulus for a few seconds, and (3) increasing doses of the avoided stimulus as the patient's calm is maintained. Operant conditioning includes a combination of (1) positive reinforcement, (2) differential reinforcement (a selected combination of positive reinforcement and extinction), (3) shaping (a specific course of reinforcement), (4) punishment, and (5) negative reinforcement. Examples of positive reinforcement are approval, an ice-cream cone, a gift certificate, and images of beautiful scenery. Examples of negative reinforcement are electric shock, drugs that induce vomiting, and horrible imagery. Other behavioral techniques are goal-setting, undoing, interrupting the impulse/action cycle, identifying cues and triggers to harmful behavior, and behavioral monitoring.

A behavioral approach is important for any patient population in which there is behavioral disturbance but it is also important to look at what behaviors any therapy is reinforcing. Are group members reinforced for coming late or early, for talking or not talking, and so on? Is the therapist using negative or positive reinforcement for certain behaviors and with what results? Even interpretations can be viewed as positive or negative reinforcement: the therapist may be seen as giving the patient attention or admonishment (e.g., "Take responsibility for your behavior!").

Secondary gains of certain behaviors often go unnoticed, causing maladaptive behavior to continue. A member may be open and tearful in group, telling others about the terrible day he had the day before and how he messed up everything from morning to night. The group is spellbound. The therapist needs to wonder here whether the member is getting secondary gain from his distress because he is getting so much attention from others for his misery. In this sense, the group is positively reinforcing his self-destructive behavior.

It is important that patients' and therapist's goals be realistic so that they can be reached and so that there can be some sense of accomplishment in reaching them (positive reinforcement). It is not uncommon for therapists working with inpatients or schizophrenics to have goals that are too high for their patients, causing everyone to be disillusioned (Lonergan, 1982). Lonergan (1982) and Yalom (1983) both write about the frequent necessity of having one goal for a single group meeting. Patients often perpetuate their negative self-image by setting goals that are too high and thus assuring failure and self-recrimination.

Habitual behavior is hard to stop, as anyone who has tried to stop smoking, drinking, or overeating knows. Behavior therapists have tried to develop techniques to help. One of these is looking for cues or triggers to certain behaviors. "Prior to getting a drink, do you turn the television on?" "Yes." "Okay, try not turning the television on." Another tool is putting distance between one's urge to smoke (or drink or overeat) and the actual action. You keep your cigarettes in the car so that you have to go to some effort to get them. Before overeating, you sit down with a paper and pencil and answer some questions: "What is the situation now? How do I feel about it? Is there another way of solving this problem?" Monitoring behavior is also important. This can be done with charts, diaries, and journals. If a therapist makes such home assignments, it is important to utilize them in the therapy. Charts may include a point system; if a patient earns a certain number of points, he gets a reward.

Analysis

Now it is time for me to look at my process notes and see what the reinforcement patterns are. What behavior are members being reinforced for? Are there secondary gains? Is the leader aware of cognitive processing of any of the group members? Is any member working on their negative thinking? Is this a subject acceptable to discuss in the group? Are any members suffering from behavioral disturbances and, therefore, in need of cognitive and behavioral monitoring? Are members using the group to test out new behaviors or share coping mechanisms?

My analysis based on the cognitive-behavioral approach is that group therapy can be beneficial because the participants can be exposed to alternative behaviors and cognitions, can use others as models, and can use the group as a lab in which to experiment with new behaviors. In the group of bulimics, members take Mary's lead and put words to their sexuality and they reinforce each other in the process. They do this by allowing time for members to talk about their sexuality and to respond with positive feedback. The therapist's interventions further reinforce; they indicate that talk about sexuality is worthy of the leader's attention. Members respond by revealing their sexual nature in a new way (Jane with her first homosexual encounter, Mary seducing her boyfriend). The leader is concerned that Jane's behavior with her roommate is defensive and therefore wants to limit the secondary gain that Jane gets from the group. Thus she does not elicit detail about Jane's encounter with her roommate.

At the same time that reinforcement is operating in the group, the leader is looking for opportunities to help the members shift their cognitions about their sexuality, aggression, and self-image. The leader challenges members' notions that homosexual and heterosexual feelings are bad and should not be talked about. The same is true for the concepts of aggression and competitive striving. But most striking is how much the leader reinforces each member as an acceptable person. The leader is succeeding in changing members' self-images from "bad and unacceptable" to "good and acceptable" by consistently conveying acceptance of members' (formerly perceived) unacceptable thoughts and behavior (the leader says it is a compliment to be the object of homosexual passion; the leader suggests that being competitive is not a big deal).

This is a group for bulimics who have the behavior disorder of bingeing and vomiting. It is important that the norms of the group include permission to discuss bulimic behavior and ways of modifying it. Positive reinforcement should occur for any progress in curtailing the behavior. In this meeting there is no focus on behavior; instead, the leader and group are focusing on the intrapsychic conflicts beneath the symptom. It is not infrequent for a bulimic group to reach this kind of processing after behavior is under control. But if the members have not reached the point of control and there is no focus in the group on the bulimic behavior, a meeting such as this one could be resistant. (I once had a patient who came to see me for compulsive overeating; she was morbidly obese. We explored her psychodynamics thoroughly. When I asked her to tell me exactly what and when she ate during the day, she begged me not to make her do it. She said, "I'll tell you anything but that.")

If the leader wanted to explore behavioral patterns, she could use Mary's dream as an entry and ask: "We never talk about people actually bingeing and throwing up in here, and yet in this dream Lilli is doing it. How are people progressing with their bulimia?" Cognitive functioning could be approached when Jane says that she felt beautiful after her roommate told her she was. The leader could ask how she felt about herself prior to this. Undoubtedly, Jane's (and other members') bulimia is caused and perpetuated by thoughts of self-deprecation and false beliefs (e.g., "If I were thinner, I would be liked more or I would be beautiful"; "The way I am now is fat and ugly"). Others in the group could give Jane realistic feedback and then group members could talk about how to alter destructive thought patterns.

CONCLUSION

The seven group theories described in this chapter can help you improve your technique in the practice of group therapy. Application of *Freud's group psychology* attunes you to the murderous rage below the surface in a group and to the power of the collective unconscious. Use of *Bion's basic assumption theory* sharpens your awareness of the unconscious agenda of the group as a whole: to be dependent on you and idealize you as a leader, to use you to fight or flee from an enemy, or to pair you (or a group member) with someone so that you can give birth to a messiah. Understanding the *group focal conflict* assists you in making group-as-a-whole interventions. If you can figure out the group's wishes and fears and how it finds solutions to these opposing forces, you will also have a better understanding of each member's internal conflicts. *Living systems theory* aids you in determining the myriad forces impinging on a therapy group and deters oversimplifying what is contributing to the group's process. It will guide you in assessing the health of the boundaries of each group member (including yourself) and of the group as a whole. *Foulkes's psychoanalysis in groups* also aids you in organizing the complexity of the therapy group. Information can be organized into four levels: current, transference, projective, and primordial. Knowledge of each level helps you apply psychoanalytic concepts such as transference and resistance to group work. *Yalom's here-and-now approach* gives you tools for working with people on their immediate transactions in the group. Such interventions are powerful because the members re-create in the moment what they do outside the group and have done in the past. The group becomes a laboratory in which interpersonal patterns are displayed and can be corrected. *Cognitive therapy* sensitizes you to negative thinking and aids you in helping your patients think more positively and constructively. *Behavior therapy* assists you with the treatment of patients who have addictions and other maladaptive behaviors. Cognitive and behavioral techniques should be integrated with group-as-a-whole techniques when treating behavior disorders.

Invariably, therapists want to know how to choose the proper theory or technique and how to decide which to use and when? This is where judgment comes in; as such, it constitutes the art of practicing group therapy. Leading a group takes some degree of confidence and ability to be creative. Remember, theories are tools, not dictators of truth. You enter the group with an armamentarium of techniques and *you* decide what to use, when to use it, and how to use it. Then you watch for the result of your intervention and make a judgment as to what the next one will be.

REFERENCES

Agazarian, Y., & Peters, R. (1981). *The visible and invisible group*. London: Routledge and Kegan Paul.

Ashbach, C., & Schermer, V. (1987). *Object relations, the self, and the group*. London: Routledge and Kegan Paul.

Beck, A. T., Rush, A. J., Shaw, R. F., & Emery, G. (1979). *Cognitive therapy of depression*. New York: Guilford Press.

Bertalanffy, L. von (1966). General system theory and psychiatry. In S. Arieti (Ed.), *American handbook of psychiatry* (pp. 705–721). New York: Basic Books.

Bion, W. (1955). *Experiences in groups*. New York: Basic Books.

Durkin, H. (1975). The development of systems theory and its implications for the theory and practice of group therapy. In C. R. Woldberg & M. L Aronson (Eds.), *Group therapy–1975* (pp. 8–20). New York: Stratton Intercontinental.

Ellis, A. (1992). Group rational-emotive and cognitive-behavior therapy. *International Journal of Group Psychotherapy, 42*(1), 63–80.

Erikson, E. (1980). Ego development and historical change: Clinical notes. In S. Scheidlinger (Ed.), *Psychoanalytic group dynamics* (189–212). New York: International Universities Press.

Foulkes, S. H. (1948). *Introduction to group-analytic psychotherapy*. London: Heinemann.

Foulkes, S. H. (1975). Group-analytic dynamics with specific reference to psychoanalytic concepts. *International Journal of Group Psychotherapy, 7*, 40–53.

Freud, S. (1921). Group psychology and the analysis of the ego. In J. Strachey (Ed. and Trans.), *The standard edition of the complete psychological works of Sigmund Freud* (Vol. 18, pp. 67–143). London: Hogarth Press, 1955.

LeBon, G. (1920). *The crowd: A study of the popular mind*. London: Fisher Unwin.

Lonergan, E. (1982). *Group intervention: How to begin and maintain groups in medical and psychiatric settings*. New York: Jason Aronson.

Lonergan, E. (1984). Eating disorder group therapy. *Newsletter of the American Anorexia and Bulimia Association,* 7(2).

Marmor, J. (1988). Psychiatry in a troubled world: The relation of clinical practice and social reality. *American Journal of Orthopsychiatry, 58*(4), 484–491.

Minuchin, S. (1978). *Psychosomatic families.* Cambridge, MA: Harvard Universities Press.

McDougall, W. (1920). *The group mind.* New York: Putnam.

Popper, K. R. (1968). *Logic of scientific discovery.* New York: Harper & Row.

Rioch, M. (1970). The work of Wilfred Bion on groups. *Psychiatry, 33*(1), 56–66.

Rutan, J. S., & Stone, W. (1993). *Psychodynamic group psychotherapy* (2nd ed.). New York: Guilford Press.

Scheidlinger, S. (Ed.). (1980). Freud's group psychology. In *Psychoanalytic group dynamics* (pp. 5–14). New York: International Universities Press.

Sullivan H. S. (1953). *The collected works of Harry Stack Sullivan.* New York: Norton.

Whitaker, D., & Lieberman, M. (1964). *Psychotherapy through group process.* New York: Atherton.

Whitman, R., & Stock, D. (1980). The group focal conflict. In S. Scheidlinger (Ed.), *Psychoanalytic group dynamics.* New York: International Universities Press.

Wolpe, J. (1982). *The practice of behavior therapy* (3rd ed.). New York: Pergamon Press.

Yalom, I. D. (1983). *Inpatient group psychotherapy.* New York: Basic Books.

Yalom, I. D. (1985). *The theory and technique of group psychotherapy* (3rd ed.). New York: Basic Books.

INDEX

Acceptance, 44, 83
Affective processes
  catharsis, 77, 84
  expression of, 101
  in group culture, 161
  interpretation and, 88–89
  in termination of group, 94
  as therapeutic focus, 84–86
AIDS, 175
Alcohol abuse, 18, 168
  twelve-step program for, 183–185
Alcoholics Anonymous, 161
  psychotherapy with, 183–185
Altruism, 44, 83, 164, 207
American Group Psychotherapy
    Association, 28
Apologies, by therapist, 116–117
Assertiveness training, 173
Assessment. *See also* Intake interview;
    Patient selection
  of group interactions in
    differentiation stage, 48–49
  group screening, 5–6, 13, 18
  for homogeneous groups, 175
  of inpatient therapy group, 165–166
  intake interview, 4–5
  LTSG interview, 13–16
  for outpatient program, 170–171
  pregroup, 37–39
  of psychological health-sickness,
    158–159
  of psychological mindedness, 22–24
  of quality of object relations, 22,
    25–27
  for referral, 171
  STIG interview, 19–20
  treatment matching, 157–158
Attendance rules, 40–41
  intervention for breaches of, 137–139
  in LTSG, 13
  open discussion of, 71
Axis I diagnoses, 22
Axis II diagnoses, 22

B

Basic assumption theory, 196–198,
    214
Biopsychosocial orientation, 6–7
Boring patient, 129–130
Bulimia, 195, 198, 199, 208, 210,
    213

C

Catharsis, 77, 83, 84, 207
Children, 18
Closed membership, 10
Cognitive-behavioral orientation, 7–8, 20, 91, 162, 209–214, 215

Cognitive processes, therapeutic
    focus on, 86–89
Commitment, 10, 41, 161
    patient anxiety and, 11–12
Communications processes, 101–102
    boring patient, 129–130
Composition of group. *See also*
    Patient selection
    decrease in group size, 154–155
    guidelines, 63
    heterogeneous versus
        homogeneous, 9–10
    in LTSG, 12–13
    negative effects of, 120
    number of patients, 10–11
    in STIG, 17–18, 21–22
    therapeutic approach and, 123–
        124
Concurrent therapies, 3
Confidentiality, 40, 65
Contracting, 63–64. *See* Preparation
    of patient
Cotherapists
    balancing activity levels of, 74
    coleadership training model, 62–
        63
    interactions, 82
    in working group, 92–93
Countertransference
    combative patient and, 133–134
    negative effects, 120–121
    prevention and management, 116–
        118
    therapeutic utility, 116
    therapist helper-type patient, 131
    types, 115–116

D

Day programs, 169–170
Difficult patients
    boring patient, 129–130
    combative patient, 133–134
    dominant patient, 127–129

    help-rejecting patient, 134–136
    silent/withdrawn patient, 125–126
    therapist helper-type, 130–133
Disruption, 12, 58
Dropouts, 40, 119–120
Duration of group, 10
    in LTSG, 13
    in STIG, 18
    treatment approach and, 93

E

Environmental concerns, 42
Existential therapy, 8

F

Feedback
    in early sessions, 67–68
    protective intervention against, 130
First session, 41–43, 65–67
Frequency of sessions, 10
    in LTSG, 13
    in STIG, 18

G

Gender-homogeneous groups, 175–
    176
Global Assessment Scale (GAS), 158,
    159
Group focal conflict theory, 198–
    200, 214
Group relations
    in Alcoholics Anonymous, 184
    common features of, 160–161, 162
    conflict between members, 50–51,
        147–149
    in differentiation stage, 47–51, 74–
        82
    domineering individual and, 127–
        129

in early sessions, 65–69
in group focal conflict theory,
198
with help-rejecting/complaining
patient, 135–136
in here-and-now approach, 207
interaction guidelines, 70
as outcome factor, 158
outside socializing, 41, 65–66,
149–152
as patient selection criterion, 171
primitive psychological processes
in, 112–115
projective identification in, 112
scapegoating in, 50, 112–114,
128, 144–147
in self-help groups, 182
stimulating interaction, 102–
103
as therapeutic factor, 89, 162–
164
Group therapy
as adjunct therapy, 3
in basic assumption theory, 196–
198
classical psychoanalytic theory
and, 193–196
in cognitive-behavioral approach,
209–214
cohesiveness in, 161–162, 207–
208
combined psychotherapy–twelve-
step program, 183–185
in group focal conflict theory,
198–200
here-and-now approach, 207–209
in living systems theory, 200–204
for moderate problems, 170–180
other-than-psychotherapy, 180–
183
psychoanalysis in groups, 204–206
for severe problems, 165–170
theory of, 190–191
treatment matching, 157–158
types of groups, 160–165

H

Health-Sickness Rating Scale, 158,
159
Here-and-now approach, 207–209,
214
Heterogeneous groups, 9–10
long-term outpatient, 177–180
short-term, 172–175
Homework assignments, 91–92,
211
Homogeneous groups, 9–10
assessment for, 175
gender-specific, 175–177
schizophrenic patients in, 167
short-term outpatient, 176–177
specialized inpatient, 168–170
Hope, 44, 83, 163–164, 207

I

Identification process, 179
Individual therapy
as concurrent therapy, 3
in early group therapy, 43
in preparation for group therapy,
37
Inpatient treatment groups, 10
evaluation criteria, 165–166
outcome indicators, 168
partial hospitalization, 169–170
for patients with severe problems,
166–170
psychodynamic approach, 167–
168
specialized, 168–169
Intake interview, 4–5
Integrated Psychotherapy Group
model, 174–175
Interpersonal relationships. *See also*
Group relations
as goal of therapy, 101
group therapy selection criteria,
2–3

Interpersonal relationships (*continued*)
  LTSG for problems in, 11, 12–13, 16
  pregroup assessment, 37–39
  in quality of object relations
    assessment, 25–26
Interpretation
  affective arousal and, 88–89
  guidelines, 87–89
  role of, 102
  in STIG, 17

L

Leaderless groups, 12, 181
Levels approach to treatment, 56–57,
    166
Living systems theory, 200–204, 214
Long-term, time-unlimited,
    supportive group psychotherapy
    (LTSG)
  cognitive assessment for, 27
  composition of group, 12
  objectives, 12
  patient selection, 13–16, 27
  preparation, 13
  structure of group, 13
  theoretical orientation, 11–12
  therapist technique, 12, 93
Long-term heterogeneous
    outpatient group, 177–180
Loss
  of group, 18
  STIG for, 16, 18
  termination of therapy as, 57–58,
    95
LTSG. *See* Long-term, time-
    unlimited, supportive group
    psychotherapy

M

Managed care, 165
Marital relations, 3

Men's groups, 176–177
Minnesota Multiphasic Personality
    Inventory (MMPI), Global
    Severity Measure, 158, 159
Mother-child dyad, 189, 190

N

Negative outcomes, 119–122

O

Object relations, 205
  assessment, 22, 25–27
  in LTSG, 11
Outcome predictors
  group behavior as, 4
  group functioning as, 158
  group participation as, 79
  individual qualities in, 4
  in inpatient group therapy, 168
  intake interview data in, 4–5
  psychological mindedness
    assessment, 23–24
  quality of object relations in, 25,
    26
  for treatment matching, 157–158
Outpatient groups, 10
  long-term heterogenous, 177–180
  for moderate problems, 171–172
  patient selection, 170–171
  short-term heterogeneous, 172–
    175
  short-term homogeneous, 175–177

P

Paranoid disorders, 3
Participation
  in early sessions, 44–45, 66–67, 68
  excessive early self-disclosure, 44–
    45, 67–68, 139–141

as outcome indicator, 79
in termination of therapy, 57
withdrawn patient, 125–126
Patient selection
assessment instruments, 26–27
criteria, 2–6, 29–30
exclusion criteria, 3–4, 16, 21,
167–168
group behavior as criterion, 4–5
group composition in, 9–10
group screening, 5–6, 13, 18
group structure and, 10–11
individual skills criteria, 3
in Integrated Psychotherapy
Group model, 174
legitimate approach, 2–3
for long-term groups, 179–180
in LTSG, 13–16
negative effects of, 119–120
objectives, 63
outcome research, 4
for outpatient group, 170–171
practice trends, 1–2, 9
in self-help groups, 182
in short-term heterogenous
groups, 172, 173
significance of, 1
in STIG, 16, 17, 19–21
theoretical orientation and, 6–8,
29
therapist factors in, 8–9
therapist training for, 28–29, 30
in twelve-step programs, 182–
183
Personality disorders, 22, 169–170
Post-traumatic stress disorder, 161
Preparation of patient
for group processes, 39–41, 58,
64
individual therapy for, 37
interpersonal focus in, 37–39
in LTSG, 13
objectives, 63–64
patient understanding of
therapeutic change, 76–77

for premature termination, 152
in screening process, 5–6
for self-help group adjunct
therapy, 183
in STIG, 18
for termination of group, 93
Projective identification, 112, 113
Psychodynamic approach
in addiction program, 169
in inpatient group, 167–168
patient selection, 20
theoretical basis, 17
Psychological Mindedness
Assessment Procedure, 22, 23–
24

Q

Quality of care, 165
Quality of Object Relations Scale,
25–27

R

Recidivism reduction, 6–8
Referrals
patient needs assessment in, 171
referral form, 5
selection for group therapy and, 5
Regression
as group phenomenon, 112, 194
management of, 113
Reinforcement of group norms, 42–
43, 66
Relaxation training, 173
Resistance, 53
in differentiation stage, 76
as group phenomenon, 104–105
to termination of group, 57, 94–
95
theoretical concept, 103–104
treatment approach, 105–107
Role playing, 91

S

Scapegoating, 50, 112–114
  intervention for, 144–147
  risk of, 128, 144
Schizophrenic patients, 167
Self-help groups, 180–182
Session length, 10, 13, 18
Short-term, time-limited,
    interpretive group therapy
    (STIG)
  cognitive assessment for, 22–27
  composition of group, 16, 17–18
  group characteristics, 21–22
  patient preparation, 18
  patient selection, 16, 17, 19–21, 27
  structure of group, 18
  theoretical orientation, 17
  therapeutic goals, 16, 17
  therapist technique, 17
Silence, 12
  withdrawn patient, 125–126
Size of group, 10–11
  mid-treatment decisions, 154–
    155
  in STIG, 18
Socializing between members, 41,
    65–66, 149–152
Society as group, 189, 190
STIG. See Short-term, time-limited,
    interpretive group therapy
Structural Analysis of Social
    Behavior, 39
Structure of group
  discussion of, 66
  in Integrated Psychotherapy
    Group model, 174–175
  in levels approach, 166
  in LTSG, 13
  to model daily life activities, 174
  patient selection and, 10–11
  short-term inpatient models, 166–
    167
  short-term outpatient program,
    172

  in specialized inpatient groups,
    168
  in STIG, 18
Substance abuse programs, 168–169
Supervisor role, 61–62
Systems theory
  group boundaries, 45
  living systems theory, 200–204

T

Termination of group
  decrease in group size and, 154–
    155
  early risk factors, 44
  planning for, 93–94
  premature, 40, 152–154
  process of, 57–58
  resistance to, 57, 94–95
  rituals for, 95–96
  therapist role, 94
Theoretical orientation
  basic assumption theory, 196–198
  classical psychoanalysis, 193–196
  cognitive-behavioral approach,
    209–214
  common features of group
    therapies, 160–161, 162, 164
  concept of change, 162
  concept of self-understanding, 86
  group focal conflict theory, 198–
    200
  group structure and, 10–11
  here-and-now approach, 204–206
  in homogeneous groups, 175
  interpersonal focus, 47–48
  living systems theory, 200–204
  in LTSG, 11–12
  patient selection and, 6–8
  psychoanalysis in groups, 204–
    206
  psychodynamic approach, 17
  in short-term outpatient group,
    173–175

in STIG, 17
utility of theory, 189–191, 215
Therapeutic alliance
  client–therapist conflict, 79–80
  in differentiation stage, 49–50,
    75–76
  in group, 58, 59, 67
  individual sessions for, 37
  with monopolizing-type patient,
    128
Therapeutic goals
  in Alcoholics Anonymous, 184
  behavioral change, 89–92
  in cognitive-behavioral approach,
    212
  in differentiation stage, 51–52
  in engagement stage, 36
  first session, 42, 66–67
  group needs, 102–103
  in homework assignments, 91
  individual needs, 101–102
  interpersonal relations as, 101
  in long-term heterogeneous
    outpatient group, 178
  in LTSG, 12
  member interaction in, 47–48
  patient selection and, 6–8
  patient understanding of change
    processes, 76–77
  self-understanding as, 86–87
  in STIG, 17
  in time-limited groups, 71–72
  in working with affect, 84
Therapeutic process. See also
    Preparation of patient
  boundary setting, 45–47, 66, 202
  challenges in, 156
  creating framework for change,
    69–74
  developmental model, 35–36, 123–
    124
  differentiation stage, 47–53, 74–
    82
  early sessions, 43–45, 65–64
  engagement stage, 36–47

excessive early self-disclosure in,
    44–45, 67–68, 139–141
  first session, 41–43, 65–67
  in group focal conflict theory,
    199
  group resistance in, 53, 104–
    105
  in here-and-now approach, 207–
    209
  in heterogeneous outpatient
    group, 177–180
  individual expression of group
    processes, 54–56
  as interpersonal learning, 162–
    164
  levels approach, 56–57, 166
  in long-term therapies, 93, 177–
    180
  member participation, 44
  negative effects of, 119–122
  nonconstructive talk in, 58–59, 69
  in partial hospitalization
    treatment, 170
  primitive group processes in,
    112–113
  psychoanalysis in groups, 204–
    206, 214
  self-help group adjunct therapy in,
    183–185
  severe problems, short-term
    inpatient models for, 166–167
  in short-term heterogenous
    groups, 173
  substance abuse inpatient group,
    168–169
  termination stage, 57–58, 93–96
  therapeutic change in, 76–79
  utility of theory in, 189–191
  working stage, 53–57, 82–84
  working with affect, 84–86
Therapist technique. See also Difficult
    patients
  action-oriented, 88–91
  addressing group resistance, 53
  attendance problems, 137–139

Therapist technique (*continued*)
  in cognitive-behavioral approach,
    210–212
  conflict between group members,
    147–149
  in confrontation, 79–80
  countertransference prevention
    and management, 116–118
  in differentiation stage, 51–53,
    75–76
  encouraging group responsibility
    for change, 78–79, 102
  in engagement stage of therapy,
    36
  in excessive early self-disclosure,
    139–141
  exploratory, 51
  exploring intrapsychic
    phenomena, 54–55, 82–84
  first session, 42–43, 65
  group developmental stage and,
    123–124
  in group resistance, 105–107
  interpretation, 87–89
  leadership, 101
  in LTSG, 12
  maintaining positive orientation,
    66–69
  management of primitive group
    processes, 113–115
  proactive, 156
  problems in, 69–70, 73–74, 119–122
  reactivating affect, 85
  reflection of affect, 85
  reinforcement of group norms,
    42–43, 44
  resolving transference, 109–112
  self-disclosure, 80–81, 126
  setting group boundaries, 47
  in short-term outpatient group,
    173–175
  socializing between members,
    147–149
  in STIG, 17
  with stuck group, 141–144

  in termination of group, 94, 95–96
  therapeutic context of, 100, 127
  in time-limited therapy, 73
  timing of intervention, 59
Time-limited therapy. *See also* Short-
    term, time-limited, interpretive
    group therapy
  heterogeneous groups, 172–173
  outpatient groups, 171–172
  for severe cases, inpatient models
    of, 166–167
  therapeutic goals in, 71–72
  therapist style in, 73
Training of therapists
  coleadership format, 62–63
  in early group sessions, 65–74
  encouraging self-disclosure in,
    80–82
  observation of sessions, 46–47
  in patient selection, 28–29
  role of experience in, 60
  role of supervisor, 61–62
  self-monitoring in, 63
  setting for, 61
Transference
  characteristics, 108–109
  in groups, 204
  in LTSG, 12
  in STIG, 17
  therapeutic significance, 107–108
  treatment approach, 109–112
  types, 108
Twelve-step programs, 162, 169, 181,
    182–183
  with psychotherapy, 183–185

U

Universality, 44, 83, 164, 207

W

Women's groups, 176

CPSIA information can be obtained
at www.ICGtesting.com
Printed in the USA
LVHW091536270119
605402LV00005B/23/P